Creative Arts in Humane Medicine

Creative Arts in Humane Medicine

Editor: Cheryl L. McLean

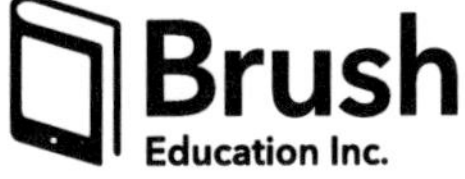

14 15 16 17 18 5 4 3 2 1

Brush Education Inc.
www.brusheducation.ca
contact@brusheducation.ca

Cover design: Carol Dragich, Dragich Design
Cover artwork: (top) *Peace of Heart* by Cyrus McEachern at cyrus.mceachern@gmail.com, from Heartfelt Images, UBC, Division of Cardiology; (bottom left) *Ventricle,* by Eva Milinkovic at tsunamiglassworks.com; (bottom right) © Dmytro Tolokonov/Veer
Copy edit: Leslie Vermeer

Printed and manufactured in Canada
Ebook edition available at Amazon, Kobo and other e-retailers.

Library and Archives Canada Cataloguing in Publication
Creative arts in humane medicine / Cheryl L. McLean, editor.
Includes bibliographical references.
Issued in print and electronic formats.
ISBN 978-1-55059-454-6 (pbk.).

1. Medicine and the humanities. 2. Arts medicine. 3. Medical care. I. McLean, Cheryl L. (Cheryl Lee), (date), editor of compilation

R702.5.C74 2013 610 C2013-903626-1 C2013-903627-X

Produced with the assistance of the Government of Alberta, Alberta Multimedia Development Fund. We also acknowledge the financial support of the Government of Canada through the Canada Book Fund for our publishing activities.

Government of Alberta

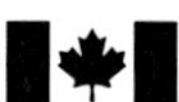

Canadian Heritage Patrimoine canadien

"Could a greater miracle take place than for us to look through each other's eyes for an instant?"

—Henry David Thoreau

Contents

Foreword

Medical Students Support Arts and Humanities in Medicine

The American Medical Student Association (AMSA)[1] has long believed that a well-rounded, nurturing medical education that supports the reflective capacity of medical students is ideal. To this end, we have a history of leadership in the humanities. It began when the Humanistic Medicine Action Committee launched the Circle of Healers institute, focusing on holistic medicine, writing and communication.

Our fourth-year elective rotation, Humanistic Elective in Alternative Medicine, Activism and Reflective Transformation, has existed for 12 years and has had physician-humanists lead its programming, among them Rachel Naomi Remen, a legend in the field and the founder of the Healers' Art curriculum. More recently, AMSA has supported the Book Discussion Webinar series, which is open to all AMSA members and features physician-authors such as Samuel Shem, Lisa Sanders and Perri Klass, to name just a few. Similarly, the Medical Humanities Scholars' Program is a semester-long, conference-call-based course that exposes 10 to 15 students to leading faculty in narrative medicine, the humanities and the arts as they explore reflective capacity, communication, self-care and the art of listening to patients' stories. Founded in 2009, this program kicked off with programming led by Rita Charon and the faculty in the narrative medicine program at Columbia University. In 2010, AMSA launched its first writers' institute, held in Washington, DC, and sponsored by the departments of humanities at Brown University School of Medicine and Stony Brook University School of Medicine.

Having personally been a part of this programming for more than six years through AMSA and in developing similar programming at my medical school, I have seen the demand for this kind of activity. After attending these events and programs, students comment that they feel re-inspired in their commitment to medicine, they have connected with their true selves as healers and they have finally found a community of like-minded physicians and physicians-in-training. AMSA believes it is paramount that the physician be not only a scientist but also a humanist, a communicator and an advocate.

—Aliye Runyan, MD
Education and Research Fellow,
American Medical Student Association

NOTE

1 The American Medical Student Association (AMSA), founded in 1950, is based in Washington, DC, and is the largest independent association of physicians-in-training in the United States. Uniquely student governed, AMSA has a membership of 68,000 from across the United States. Among its key goals are advocating for quality and affordable health care for all, equality in global health and enriching medicine through diversity.

Acknowledgments

This book has been over a year in the making, and through the process I have been privileged to work with international leaders and innovators in the field of arts and medicine; physicians; and medical educators, researchers, allied health professionals and internationally renowned artists. I want to thank each of these outstanding contributors for so generously sharing their research and educational experience with us in this volume. I am particularly inspired by the overwhelming support from medical students and residents active in arts and medicine across North America, physicians of the future expressing with conviction the belief that a well-rounded education including the arts is vital for a more humane and caring approach to medicine and quality of care.

I have also been fortunate to work with some of the best editors in the Canadian publishing industry, among them Brush Education managing editor Lauri Seidlitz and copy editor par excellence Leslie Vermeer. Thanks as well to colleague and friend Dr. Robert Kelly, a leader in the field of creativity in education in Canada, for his editing assistance and ongoing support and advice as yet another book about creative arts in interdisciplinary research advanced from concept to reality.

—Cheryl L. McLean

Introduction

Touching the Heart of What It Is To Be Human

Cheryl L. McLean

> I want to be loved with a love that is true and is truthfully expressed. I want to be loved with a love that connects me to another and connects another to me. I want to be loved with a love that embraces and that, while holding me in care, also frees me to live with care.
>
> —*John J. Guiney Yallop*

Creative Arts in Humane Medicine has been created as a resource book for medical educators, practitioners and students, as well as for those in the allied health professions who wish to learn how the arts can contribute to a more caring and empathic approach to medicine. In this collection, which features the latest research and real-life examples, physicians, medical educators, researchers and allied health professionals, as well as medical students, residents, artists and others across Canada, the United States, the United Kingdom and Australia, show how the arts in action can contribute toward humane medicine.

To be *humane* is to show empathy or understanding, to care about the condition and suffering of others, to treat others as we ourselves might wish to be treated. The word *medicine*, from the Latin *ars medicina*, refers to the art of healing, the practice invested in the treatment and prevention of illness. Humanistic medicine is a growing trend today as more medical professionals integrate the arts into their practice to improve communication with their patients and build better relationships. A recent study found that more than half the medical schools in the United States involved the arts in some form in learning activities (Rodenhauser, Strickland & Gambala, 2004). This survey showed that the arts are being used to foster student well-being, enhance teaching and learning, and improve clinical and relational skills: observation and diagnostic skills, reflection and insight, for example.

There are other encouraging signs that the arts are alive and thriving in medical education today, with programs integrating the arts and humanities into medical education and leading medical schools and universities offering more programming to promote creative and scholarly work at the intersections of the arts, humanities and medicine. One Canadian effort, the Medical Humanities HEALS (Healing and Education Through the Arts and Life Skills) Program at the Faculty of Medicine, Dalhousie University, offers programming in visual arts, performing arts, the history of medicine and creative writing. Another—the Arts and Humanities in Health and Medicine Program at the Faculty of Medicine and Dentistry, University of Alberta, launched in May 2006—has a mandate to balance scientific knowledge and compassionate care. Its mission statement formally acknowledges "the explicit recognition within the Faculty that clinical practice is both an art and a science." At the University of Toronto, the Undergraduate Medical Education (UME) program has begun to integrate different types of narrative systematically into the curriculum with a new companion curriculum.

At Yale School of Medicine, the Yale Medical Humanities and the Arts Council reports it is committed to fostering the use of the humanities, the social sciences and the arts as lenses for examining issues in health, medicine and healing. Arts and Humanities at Harvard Medical School aims to promote the role of the humanities in medical education, clinical care and research. At Stanford School of Medicine, the Arts, Humanities and Medicine program has been established to promote creative and scholarly work at the intersections among these disciplines.

Growing support for the creative arts in humane medicine today is also coming from medical students themselves. The American Medical Student Association (AMSA) has more than 150 chapters in medical schools across the United States and an estimated 350 pre-med chapters. Aliye Runyan, MD, Education and Research Fellow, American Medical Student Association, reports that the AMSA Medical Humanities Scholars program exposes students to leading faculty in narrative medicine, the humanities and the arts as they explore reflective capacity, communication, self-care and the art of listening to their patients' stories. AMSA, Runyan writes, "believes it is paramount that the physician not only be a scientist but a humanist, a communicator and an advocate."

I was recently a guest presenter for AMSA's Medical Humanities Scholars program. During the session a student asked, "If this work [about the creative arts in medicine] is frequently about empathy and feeling the human story, how much empathy is too much empathy? What if I can no longer bear it?"

The student asked a very difficult question, one not easy to answer. Our creative work is powerful and profound in the way it frequently uses all the senses to foster empathy and draw us closer to human understanding. But what *are* our human limits? I asked myself, if I were in bed, ill and fighting for life, how much empathy would I hope my caregivers would extend to me? When would enough be enough? This collection raises provocative questions and proposes alternative approaches in the hopes of inspiring new areas of investigation while opening up a larger conversation about the creative arts in medicine among students and medical practitioners.

This book has been divided into four distinct and related sections: Section 1, Educating for Empathy Through the Arts; Section 2, The Arts and Practitioner Self-Care; Section 3, Navigating with Narrative Through Life Experience; and Section 4, The Creative Arts in Action for Change in Health.

Section 1 opens with special attention to the overriding theme in this collection, that of fostering empathy through a variety of arts methodologies. We begin with visual art as the focus. André Smith and his research team at the Department of Sociology, University of Victoria, demonstrate an innovative pedagogical approach using fabric art to teach empathy with end-of-life health care providers. Similarly, in my article, I share the process of creating an ethnodrama to raise awareness about aging, mental health and autonomy, and discuss how writing and creating a performance based on research led to greater empathy and human understanding. Craig Chen, MD, an anesthesiology resident at Stanford University Medical Centre, supports the view that the arts and humanities can bring about understanding about illness and disease. In his essay he explains,

> It is not easy to go to work every day and care for people who hurt themselves, are going to die, cry on your shoulder, feel terrified or distrust the health care system. With respect to medicine, the arts and humanities help us understand how humans experience illness and disease, and place that experience in a context of diagnosis, treatment and care.

The section's closing paper, by researchers Mina Borromeo, Heather Gaunt and Neville Chiavaroli from the Melbourne Dental School, explores the visual arts used in education for increasing observational skills and understanding as students are guided through the rediscovery and re-appreciation of human responses as it applies to special-needs dentistry.

In Section 2, we examine the daily realities of working in medicine—illness, disease, aging, death and after death—and how the arts can offer healthy opportunities for practitioners to address their self-care needs. Alim Nagji, MD, who is also an actor, producer and writer, stresses that teaching practitioners to understand their patients' stories must begin early in training, before the erosion of empathy. Nagji believes using theatre in medical education can help students delve into patients' back stories, drawing parallels between those experiences and students' own. In Maura McIntyre's article, arts-informed research, part of the growing genre of performance ethnography, offers caregivers and others an opportunity to participate in reader's theatre so that they might experience real stories of nursing home life. Craig Chen informs us about the importance of providing health professionals and others a place for self-expression through varied forms of performance. At Stanford, medical students and community members connected through performance while audiences learned more about what it is like to work in the field of anesthesiology. Rachael Allen, an artist in residence at university anatomy and clinical skills laboratories in northeast England, writes about witnessing students engaged in lab work with prepared prosections of embalmed and plastinated specimens. She believes it is fundamentally important for health and humane medicine that students working in anatomy labs are offered opportunities to express these intimate human encounters through art. Allen offers new and sensory approaches to anatomy and clinical studies while artistically rendering the undergraduate experiences of medical students. Music therapy, too, has long been recognized as an effective tool for self-expression and healing and, as Amy Clements-Cortés demonstrates in her article, can also help address stress and other issues for those working in palliative care settings. In other programs, expressive approaches have also proven useful for health care practitioners, as Diane Kaufman, MD, and her team at the University of Medicine and Dentistry of New Jersey explain.

Readers will explore personal stories through narrative in Section 3 as well as learning about the applications of literature in medical practice. Each of our contributors navigates with narrative or uses story in unique ways, but all writers in this section share an underlying belief about the humanity and dignity that can be found through fostering the practitioner–patient relationship. Jasna Schwind, a nurse educator, writes about her work, informed by narrative inquiry, while sharing aspects of her own illness story to demonstrate how intentional and thoughtful reflection allowed her, as both patient and caregiver, to make sense of the experience. Narrative and poetic inquirer John J. Guiney Yallop writes about his lived experiences with medical practitioners over time and, in so doing, poignantly illustrates the importance of the relationship between practitioner and patient. Catherine L. Mah, a scientist, practitioner, researcher and teacher, discusses the uses of literature and the childhood novel in pediatrics practice, suggesting the approach may help establish a foundation for narrative examination in the one on one interview.

In Section 4 we embrace change and the future, opening with an exploration by Louise Younie, a clinical senior lecturer, who writes about her journey of discovery through arts-based inquiry and considers the transformative influences of the arts in medical education as well as within her own work. Canadian activist artists Carole Condé and Karl Beveridge are featured demonstrating the arts in action for change: the power of story and photography to touch people and advocate for humanity for those who work in health care settings. Bandy X. Lee, MD, believes there is a great need for collective and emotional healing today. She reports that, in terms of change, effective violence prevention may be the key to health and human flourishing and creativity. Louise Terry illustrates how digital stories and technology can help teach ethics and law to health and social service professionals while contributing to humane medicine. Visual and audio technologies, she suggests, help bring to life our human stories complete with actions, omissions, aspirations and values. Carol Ann Courneya closes this section with an exhibit from the heart as medical and fine arts students from the University of British Columbia build bridges to understanding health and the heart while connecting to communities through the visual arts.

This is an educational book in which, through creative processes, we feel the human story and touch the heart of what it is to be human in others while attentively loving and caring for ourselves … not only surviving but thriving as humane practitioners in our lives and work. I invite you, through this book, to read, engage and actively learn about the creative arts in humane medicine. I believe you will find, in keeping with the embodied nature of our field, each article unfolds in its way as a story, a revealing performance about life, a creative act in itself.

SECTION 1
EDUCATING FOR EMPATHY THROUGH THE ARTS

1

Teaching Empathy Through Role-Play and Fabric Art

An Innovative Pedagogical Approach for End-of-Life Health Care Providers

André Smith, Jane Gair, Phyllis McGee, Janice Valdez and Peter Kirk, MD

This chapter explores the experiences of first- and second-year medical students who participated in a learning intervention that used fabric art and role-playing to foster the acquisition of empathy skills for end-of-life care. The intervention centers on students' engagement with artwork by renowned artist Deidre Scherer, who depicts the processes of aging, dying and grieving in her work. We collected data from qualitative interviews with students and from observations of students' participation in the intervention. The students reported experiencing intense feelings of empathy toward the patients depicted in the artwork. Based on these experiences, they successfully formulated empathetic responses that took into account the imagined perspectives of these patients. We conclude that this learning intervention effectively cultivated empathy in the students who took part in the study.

Introduction

Caring for elderly individuals who are dying constitutes a pivotal but often largely unacknowledged aspect of the health care system. Given increases in life expectancy and the proliferation of life-prolonging treatments, the majority of deaths now occur in old age and take place in hospital or long-term care facilities (Northcott & Wilson, 2008). Palliative care in such settings focuses on reducing pain and discomfort rather than on halting or delaying the progress of disease (World Health Organization, 2007). Because older adults often experience vulnerable states, health care providers also find themselves needing to respond to older patients' emotional needs (Roter et al., 1997; Halpern, 2003; Shapiro & Hunt, 2003; Larson & Yao, 2005). Being empathetic under such circumstances may prove demanding for health care providers, but it can also yield important benefits for patients' quality of end-of-life care. Research on empathy in the clinical relationship suggests considerable benefits that may transfer to the context of palliative care. For example, empathetic physicians are more successful at making patients adhere to prescribed drug treatments, thus improving therapeutic outcomes such as pain management (Piette, Heisler, Krein & Kerr, 2005). Empathetic physicians also elicit more complete medical histories from their patients, thus improving diagnostic accuracy and treatment decisions (Halpern, 2003; Larson & Yao, 2005). In addition, they are less likely to be sued for malpractice (Meryn, 1998) and more likely to be perceived as trustworthy (Butow, Maclean, Dunn, Tattersall & Boyer, 1997). Finally, empathetic physicians report high levels of professional satisfaction, derive more meaning from their work and are less likely to experience burnout, which is a constant concern in palliative care (Roter et al., 1997).

Unfortunately, health care providers are often ill equipped to address the psychosocial needs of older dying patients and their families, in part because the teaching of empathetic skills is underdeveloped in medical and paramedical curricula (Halpern, 2001; Price, 2004; Nordgren & Olsson, 2004). As Kidd and Connor (2008) found in their survey of medical humanities and arts-based activities across Canada, instructors in medical humanities feel their field is marginalized in Canadian medical schools partly because instruction tends to be voluntary and rarely extends beyond the pre-clinical years. Another reason is that medical education tends to privilege scientific knowledge of body systems and diagnostics at the expense of interpersonal skills and psychological awareness (Starr, 1982; Wilkes, Milgrom & Hoffman, 2002).[1] Yet, as Garden (2007) remarks, "learning about the way an individual patient experiences and makes meaning from illness and the social context of that suffering is vastly different from the way students are tested on knowledge about the organ systems and disease" (p. 564). As a result, health care providers learn to manage patients' physical symptoms systematically and efficiently but tend to neglect the existential and experiential aspects associated with death and dying (Kirk, 2011).

Teaching Empathy: A Brief Survey of the Literature

A strong proponent of improving empathy training in medicine is Jodi Halpern, a psychiatrist, a philosopher and Professor of Bioethics and Medical Humanities at the University of California, Berkeley. In *From detached concern to empathy: Humanizing medical practice* (2001), Halpern rejects outdated notions of scientific objectivity that discourage empathy training and claims that "empathy requires experiential, not just theoretical, knowing" (p. 72). According to Halpern, learning to be empathetic requires physicians to "imagine how it feels to experience something, in contrast to imagining that something is the case" (p. 85). Unfortunately, existing programs that teach empathy typically lack the sophistication needed to reflect Halpern's pedagogical vision. Students learn about empathy primarily in the classroom, although evidence suggests that experiential learning (e.g., modeling the responses of an empathetic mentor in a clinical setting) is more effective (Henry-Tillman, Deloney, Savidge, Graham & Klimberg, 2002; Larson & Yao, 2005; Stepien & Baernstein, 2006). Didactic approaches to teaching empathy are also less effective in securing students' enthusiastic participation than alternate approaches, such as viewing a painting depicting illness or engaging in role-playing (Hoffman, Brand, Beatty & Hamill, 1985; Wikström, 2003).

Recognizing the limitations of didactic teaching methods, researchers over the past two decades have developed pedagogical approaches centred on the use of "works of narrative, the visual arts, anthropology, history, and journalism [to] encourage reflection and critical thinking about the human body and mind" (Kidd & Connor, 2008, p. 47). These researchers argue that including the medical humanities in medical and paramedical curricula can serve a corrective role for the reductionism of biomedicine and contribute to the training of reflective practitioners with an empathic understanding of the patient (Bleakley, Marshall & Brömer, 2006; DasGupta & Charon, 2004; Ousager & Johannessen, 2010). Students' reading of literature or reflecting on paintings that depict illness circumstances can enhance their understanding of the doctor–patient relationship and their ability to express themselves in non-technical language (e.g., Calman & Downie, 1996; Calman, 2001; Elizur & Rosenheim, 1982; McManus, 1995; Moyle, Barnard & Turner, 1995; Stowe & Igo, 1996; Smith, 1998; Skelton, Macleod & Thomas, 2000). For example, in one pedagogical intervention, fourth-year medical students learned to care for patients in a more humane and thoughtful manner during a one-month humanities elective (Anderson & Schiedermayer, 2003). This intervention combined an artist presenting drawings of a cancer patient, a teacher leading a tour of an art museum and a discussion of selected readings. The students kept journals and were asked to write a poem and either an essay or a short story. Similar pedagogical interventions were successfully used with medical residents (Barnard, 1994; Risse, 1992) and nurses and midwives (Begley, 1996; Castledine, 1998). Several studies report similar success in engaging students to assess the experiences, feelings and activities of ill individuals depicted in artwork (e.g., Brett-MacLean & Yiu, 2006; Blomqvist, Pitkälä & Routasalo, 2007; Wikström, 2001). Medical students taking part in art-appreciation classes significantly improved their observational skills (Bardes, Gillers & Herman, 2001; Dolev, Friedlaender & Braverman, 2001), and at least one study reports that students considered their personal and professional development to be enhanced by studying the arts (Lazarus & Rosslyn, 2003).

Another pedagogical innovation in empathy education involves the use of theatre performance and role-playing (Shapiro & Hunt, 2003). Theatre performance provides opportunities for students to identify with imagined roles and situations as either viewers or participants. This process can prove effective in fostering empathy by requiring health care providers to take on a patient's point of view in seeking to understand his/her illness circumstances (DeVito, 1999). In this manner, theatre performance can foster deeper understanding of the interactional dynamics involved in a caring and empathetic relationship (Lewis & Johnson, 2000; Welch & Welch, 2008). One example that illustrates this process is Deloney and Graham's (2003) study in which first-year medical students viewed Margaret Edson's Pulitzer Prize–winning play *Wit* as part of an experiential learning module. The play relates the personal story of a patient dying from ovarian cancer and depicts her experiences of medical care from diagnosis to death. Surveying students' responses after they had viewed *Wit*, the authors concluded that the play improved students' empathy and understanding of the lived experience of end-of-life care.

Role-playing can similarly allow students to imagine illness from the patient's perspective (Booth, 2003). More specifically, performing a dramatic role can engage students in empathetic reasoning by requiring they put themselves in another person's psychological frame of reference and imagine that person's thoughts, feelings and behaviours, which are important aspects of empathic communication (Suchman,

Markakis, Beckman & Frankel, 1997). For this reason, role-playing represents an effective experiential technique for developing empathy skills (Bolton, 1984), a view confirmed by several studies of this technique (Deeney, Johnson, Boore, Leyden & McCaughan, 2001; Ekebergh, Lepp & Dahlberg, 2004; Wasylko & Stickley, 2003).

Description of the Teaching Intervention

Despite the advent of innovative empathy pedagogies, researchers have paid little attention to their potential usefulness in teaching empathy skills to providers of end-of-life elder care. Our pilot study addresses this gap in knowledge with a unique approach that combines appreciation of fabric art and role-playing techniques adapted from drama therapy (see Bolton, 1984). Our aim is to investigate how combining fabric-art appreciation and role-playing can help students empathize with older patients at the end of life. For this reason, we planned the study to coincide with an exhibit at the University of Victoria's Maltwood Art Museum and Gallery by well-known American fabric artist Deidre Scherer (1998). Scherer has been praised for the honesty and respect with which she explores the processes of aging, dying and grieving. She addresses issues of aging and mortality by building a series of images based on elders and mentors in her community, drawing her inspiration from actual situations and models in hospices and nursing homes.

The exhibit featured 15 fabric scenes depicting end-of-life scenarios among patients and their loved ones. One series, *Surrounded by family and friends*, consisted of six life-sized scenes involving intergenerational and non-traditional families from culturally diverse groups. The other series, *The last year*, featured nine scenes documenting the final year in an elderly woman's life.[2] Using cotton, linen and silk, Scherer combines the techniques of cutting, layering and machine stitching to lend a narrative quality to her scenes. She also draws on other art-media techniques, including painting, collage, portraiture, quilting, mosaic and stained glass.

Our intervention's role-playing component involved asking students to take on alternate roles of physician and patient. A learning facilitator trained in drama therapy (J. Valdez) asked participants to focus on selected scenes from Scherer's work and to imagine how patients in those scenes would feel about their circumstances. We also used role-playing to help participants imagine how, as physicians, they would establish a therapeutic alliance and understand the circumstances of their patients' illnesses (Stepien & Baernstein, 2006). This goal of this technique was to help students acquire the "ability to understand the patient's inner experiences and perspective and a capability to communicate this understanding" (Hojat et al., 2002, p. 1563).[3] Next, we asked students once again to assume the role of care provider and think of how they would respond using specific communicative strategies (e.g., comfort, reassurance) and language to express their feelings and understandings of the imagined concerns of the patients (Charon, 2001; Morse, Bottorff, Anderson, O'Brien & Solberg, 1992).

Methods

Five medical students from the University of British Columbia's Island Medical Program, based at the University of Victoria, volunteered for the study after attending an information session open to all students in the program. We introduced the study as an investigation of how art could improve empathy and communication skills between physicians and patients. The criteria for inclusion in the study were full-time enrolment in the Island Medical Program and a willingness to participate in an intervention involving the arts. The sample included one first-year student and four second-year students; four students were female and one was male. The mean age was 26 years. This sample was drawn from a pool of 24 first-year and 24 second-year students. The ratio of male to female students in this pool was approximately 50:50.

We are aware that this sample is too small to make generalizable claims about the intervention and that it is skewed toward female second-year students. Obtaining generalizable results from this intervention would require a different research design with a larger sample of students who could be assigned to either an intervention or a control group. Such a study would also involve the use of standardized measures of empathy before and after the intervention—and, ideally, several times afterwards to measure the intervention's lasting effects. However, such a design is ill suited for the in-depth exploration of students' learning experiences that interested us in this pilot study. A quantitative quasi-experimental study will constitute a subsequent step in investigating the effectiveness and applicability of this intervention.

Our design is inspired by the principles of phenomenographic research, a widely used qualitative approach in the field of higher-education research. *Phenomenography* "is an empirically based approach that aims to identify the qualitatively different ways in which different people experience, conceptualize, perceive and understand various kinds of phenomena" (Richardson, 1999, p. 53).[4] Within such a framework, learning is conceptualized as a qualitative change from one conception about some particular aspect of reality to another conception of reality (Marton, 1988). In phenomenography, researchers aim to describe variations in how people understand a particular phenomenon (Johansson, Marton & Svensson, 1985). To achieve this aim, researchers systematically explore participants' experiences, classifying them into categories according to their similarities and differences (Marton & Pong, 2005). This approach is compatible with two key concepts in learning and teaching empathy: learning empathy as a process of understanding suffering from the patient's perspective, and teaching empathy as a process of engaging the patient's experiences in a critical and reflexive manner.

Sample size in phenomenographic research varies depending on the phenomenon's complexity. For studying broad and complex phenomena, a sample size of between 15 and 20 is considered sufficiently large to reveal variations in viewpoints (Trigwell, 2000). However, for a more circumscribed phenomenon such as this intervention, a smaller sample size is considered adequate. Although we desired a slightly larger sample size for this study, the small number of participants we recruited nevertheless yielded rich enough data to provide useful insights into the various experiences and benefits of our intervention.

Data Collection

A brief interview with students before the intervention allowed us to familiarize ourselves with their views on empathy in the physician–patient relationship. After the intervention, we interviewed students about their learning experiences, their reactions to the fabric artwork, how they felt the exercises helped them to formulate empathetic responses and how peer-to-peer interactions and the group session facilitated their learning. We collected further data by observing students during the intervention.

All interviews were audio recorded and transcribed verbatim for analysis by the investigators, according to the principles of phenomenographic research. We read the transcribed interviews to identify significant statements related to the phenomenon of learning empathy. These statements were grouped into themes, themes into clusters and clusters into categories on the basis of shared meaning (Spencer, Ritchie & O'Connor, 2003). At several points during the process, we assessed the findings' trustworthiness by having two investigators code transcripts independently and comparing the significant statements they independently identified. Consistent inter-investigator agreement obtained on these comparisons indicates good trustworthiness for our analysis. Because participants came from a tightly knit cohort of medical students, we determined that the best way to protect their anonymity was to remove all identifying information from the narrative account. Because the study had only one male student, we also decided to use the gender-neutral term *student* instead of pseudonyms as a further measure to protect anonymity.

Findings

Effective teaching of empathy is facilitated by students having a baseline understanding of why empathy is important. If they do not value empathy, they will not likely be motivated to learn about it. Learning empathy occurs more effectively when students having some basic conceptual understanding of empathy as a human response and can connect learning with their own real-life experiences (Bereiter, 1992; Bereiter & Scardamalia, 1996). If students lack a notion of what empathy entails in practical terms, trying to teach them specific skills for empathizing with patients will likely present significant challenges. However, as Morse et al. (1992) note, students typically begin their training by equating empathy with alternative responses (e.g., sympathy, pity and commiseration), which are judged non-beneficial or even harmful in the clinical setting. The goal of empathy training is therefore to teach students empathy strategies that allow them to solve practical issues in the patient–physician relationship—such skills involve controlled emotive engagement and communication that address and respond to the specific needs and concerns of patients (Morse et al., 1992).

On this basis, we conducted baseline interviews before the intervention to determine whether or not students met these necessary preconditions for effective empathy teaching. The results from these interviews confirmed that students perceived empathy as a valuable feature of the patient–physician relationship, although their responses understandably indicated vagueness in their conceptualization of empathy as clinical practice. One student remarked, "The physician must have compassion and a high level of empathy in relating to what the patient is experiencing"; another student said, "I think the physician has to be able to understand their patients, where they are coming from, what their fears, their hopes are." In addition, students commented on the importance of "intuition" in determining how best to address the concerns and emotional needs of their patients:

> We also have to be very intuitive ... know how to take what they are saying and understand what they are really saying, or what they are leaving out and what they are saying because they think they should be saying that.

Finally, students emphasized the role of reflexivity in empathetic communication, with one student commenting,

> I think it is important to be thoughtful and reflective as a physician. If you can't reflect on your own experiences and your own prejudices and opinions about things then you probably won't be able to identify issues in your own interactions with the patients.

Another student articulated how one's own life experiences with loss and grief could enhance one's ability to understand the needs of suffering and dying patients:

> I can relate to suffering because I have suffered. If you are in touch with your emotions and know what that is like, you can identify with someone in a similar situation and know what it feels like to want to be comforted and wanting to have that suffering relieved.

Students also critiqued the inadequate instruction about empathy they received in problem-based learning (PBL) lectures, a venue "not really meant for empathy," which they described as better suited to the "nuts and bolts of physiology." As one student succinctly remarked, "Having someone tell you about empathy is a lot different than feeling empathy." Students expressed a desire to learn experientially—by observing preceptors with an empathetic predisposition, for example. As one student noted, "There is just something about strong role models that gives you a feeling that you would want to imitate; an inspiration that gives you the drive to learn better skills."

Overall, these students valued empathy as an important aspect of the patient–physician relationship. The students also had some personal experiences that gave them grounds for conceptualizing empathy in the context of palliative care. They were motivated to learn empathy skills and appreciated the opportunity to do so—an opportunity they felt their medical training had thus far denied them. Our findings about students' valorization of empathy are not unexpected: several studies report that first- and second-year medical students generally begin their education valuing empathy but that empathetic concern for patients drops as their education progresses, an effect that is especially marked during their residency (Bellini, Baime & Shea, 2002; Newton et al., 2000; Wolf, Balson, Faucett & Randall, 1989).

Having ascertained students' receptiveness to empathy training, we then focused on helping them acquire more specific skills in the context of palliative care. In the next section, we report on the students' experiences with this intervention, for which we coined the acronym REAL (Reflecting and Engaging with the Arts to Learn).

Reflecting and Engaging with the Arts

The first stage of the intervention was designed to encourage students to imagine vividly the circumstances of adults depicted at the end of life. In the first exercise, the facilitator asked the students to walk around the art gallery, to reflect on the various scenes depicted in the fabric artwork, to note their reactions and to share these reactions with one another. One student described the evocative nature of the artwork in this way:

> It was going to a place in my mind that I don't know if I could have gone to without having an image to take me there. It was connecting to a moment of someone's life, or the end of their life. Through art is a really interesting way to do it, rather than having a real patient in front of you. Just to tell a story about someone in that moment I don't think could be as powerful as actually seeing the image.

When asked to elaborate on these emotional reactions, the students said they were touched by the vivid colours and varied fabric textures of the artwork. These comments were typical: "A lot of the colours and the tones and the images added to the emotion of them. They could really strike something inside that just made you connect to what that person, or that image, was experiencing at that moment." Another student added, "I felt very strongly that they were real people who I was looking at, who had something to say." Another student specifically remarked on how the artwork helped facilitate empathetic engagement with the troubling circumstances of death and dying:

> There was a catalyst to trigger emotions with the art. We have had a lot of lectures on palliative care, but they have been really dry and almost superficial about how to manage patients. But the art kind of gets right to that level of emotion, where there are a lot of things that are happening at that present moment. I felt it was a connection with that.

These comments suggest the artwork's effectiveness in helping students transpose the represented illness circumstances into vividly experienced internal emotions.

In the next phase of the intervention, the facilitator engaged the students in role-playing. This technique required students to select a patient from one of the scenes and to begin imagining what that patient was experiencing. The intention was to prompt students to imagine the patient's perspective before responding empathetically to the patient's concerns. Students did indeed find this technique valuable in helping them appreciate the unique circumstances of the patients depicted in the artwork, as this comment makes clear:

> It was just nice to just think about the feelings of the people in the pictures, their situation. There was an interesting picture called *At Night*. It was an elderly man,

> and it just showed his face and it was at night. I hadn't thought about that before, about nighttime being such a difficult time for these patients and what we can we do for them during this time. Because often sleep is disrupted, and if you wake up and no one is around, it is really lonely.

Another student spoke about gaining a better grasp of end-of-life care as a lived experience:

> I guess the sadness just comes from knowing that these people are inside. Like looking at people inside, and feeling empathy for them. I can think of certain women in those pictures just looking at me, and feeling "Oh, it must be really hard to be you." It is almost like they were saying, this is what my life is, and I felt that I was communicating with them.

One student felt attuned to the patients' despair: "They were lonely. I felt they were alone, a hopeless situation," while another remarked, "With making a story about the person, it became about the family member. It was really close to me. So it was feelings associated with thinking about my own death or about the death of people that are close to me."

In the next phase, the facilitator asked students to assume the role of the physician comforting that patient. This time, we intended to give students the opportunity to consider how they would express empathy in the context of end-of-life care. In this exercise, students were asked to focus their attention on strategies that would address the specific needs and concerns of the patients in the artwork. Students identified several useful techniques, including "taking your time to listen to the patient," "being with the patient" and "not imposing your feelings on the patient's care." Students also learned to develop strategies based on what they would expect others to do for them if they themselves were patients, as illustrated by the following comment:

> I would want to receive news not with my family. But that comes from me not being a person who likes to share emotion. If somebody is really emotional, it depends on the circumstances. But I would want to deal with it myself and then face my family or my friends. I don't know for sure if I would [want] to do that. I guess I am clearer on how I would feel than on what I would do.

As part of this exercise, the facilitator asked students to imagine a life history for a patient of their choice (including details about the patient's family life, work history and hobbies) and to speculate about how these details would affect the patient's experience of palliative care. This exercise helped students to humanize patients as individuals with unique biographies beyond their medical histories. In reflecting on this exercise, one student astutely remarked,

Being a physician means being around a lot of patients all the time and I wonder if a lot of doctors do feel that after a while they become desensitized to death or to the patients. They see a lot of older dying patients as the same. But I think it is important to remember that every one of them has had a full life and that they are someone's mother or someone's father and to make sure that every patient remains kind of a human with a whole story to them.

Group Debriefing and Post-Intervention Interviews

In the final stage of the intervention, the students participated in a group debriefing session in which they shared their learning experiences, their views on empathy, death and dying and their concerns about communicating empathy in the context of challenging end-of-life scenarios. We included this group session in the intervention because research suggests that peer-to-peer interactions can help practitioners learn from one another how best to respond to patients in the sensitive situations often encountered in palliative care (Elizur & Rosenheim, 1982; Lancaster, Hart & Gardner, 2002).

The students credited the group session for helping them appreciate the diverse ways of responding to patients with empathy. As one student revealed,

I could just see that they had picked up on different things from the art, and what we saw wasn't tied to art only but also to history and our own experiences with death and our own natural feelings of it. So that helped me to understand how they saw death differently than I did.

Students also appreciated the trust that developed in the group, expressing how this trust allowed them to disclose personal thoughts and feelings:

It is kind of liberating to share what you are feeling with others [and] really valuable to be vulnerable with them. That is not something that we get to do very much and I would really like to do that more often, because I think it really changes my attitudes about other people. I felt that I got to be closer to them for doing it.

Other students added that the competitive climate of medical school discouraged them from engaging in such supportive exchanges. Participants also appreciated that the group session allowed them to forge a sense of community among themselves as learners and future health care providers. Participants felt that medical practitioners would benefit from taking part in such an intervention, regardless of their appreciation for the arts:

I think that everyone should have to do it if they are going to be practicing medicine. Even if it makes them uncomfortable, you have to face it if you are going

> to be in medicine, whether you are doing palliative care or not. I don't think that anyone would lose anything.

In reflecting on their learning experiences in post-intervention interviews, the students lauded the intervention for providing them with specific ways to assess the personal dimensions of patients' end-of-life needs. This approach proved a welcome counterpoint to the diagnostic emphasis that typically characterizes patient–physician encounters. As one student remarked, "You start to lose focus, you do other things, and I think it is really good to just redirect your attention every once in a while. I think that is more what it has done for me." Another student similarly underlined, "Being competent is more than just focusing on the relevant details and science and I think this is one way of just bringing me back to the bigger picture." Finally, one student expressed how the type of experiential learning fostered by the intervention could translate into life-long self-exploration:

> I really enjoyed the process and I think in the future it will probably give me another method of processing things. I hope that, if I have time in my life where I need to think more about a certain subject, that maybe I will consider using art to do that.

Overall, the students reported the intervention to be effective in enhancing their awareness of the palliative-care circumstances depicted in the artwork. They also considered the guided reflection and role-play exercises to be instrumental in helping them develop skills in formulating empathetic responses that were specifically geared toward the needs and concerns of patients at end of life.

Discussion

Death and dying constitute difficult aspects of medical care, particularly in the context of geriatric care. End of life introduces unique challenges for health care providers: they must not only care for patients' physical health but also grapple with patients' and families' emotional pain—and with patients' and families' unresolved issues. Such emotional issues often pose as communication barriers between patients and health care providers. While health care providers likely enter their discipline favourably predisposed to empathy, they do not necessarily possess the specific empathy skills needed to manage patient encounters effectively, particularly in challenging palliative-care scenarios. Current clinical training poorly prepares providers to deal with these kinds of scenarios where treatment options are few and empathetic communication is crucial in fostering quality care (Dickinson, 2007). Without proper training, providers may later resort to coping strategies such as distancing themselves emotionally from their patients (Ross, 1978).

Yet, as Halpern (2001) argues, medical judgment cannot be based on such complete detachment—rather, some level emotional engagement can enable health care providers to understand more completely the "particular meanings that a symptom or a diagnosis has for an individual" (p. 40). Our intervention provides an initial step to empower health care providers with emotional sensitivity to older adults at end of life. We sought to centre students' learning on the palliative-care circumstances depicted in the artwork and prompted them to construct their own responses to these circumstances. The guided reflection and role-playing exercises gave them an opportunity to learn to manage their own emotions while appraising patients' circumstances. We also encouraged students to share and examine one another's responses in an effort to foster learning as a co-operative knowledge-building experience.

Our findings also underscore the value of combining art appreciation with role-playing techniques. Deidre Scherer's fabric art lends itself well to this type of intervention: reviewers of Scherer's work have commented on her ability to use fabric art to express profound human emotions, imbuing her subjects with a sense of human presence and representing grief and love in a powerful manner. As Cohen (2001) remarks, "the viewer is swept into the scene. One only pulls back to marvel at her technical mastery and the surprise that the medium is fabric and not acrylic or oil paint" (p. 2524). The aesthetic qualities of the fabric artwork are therefore crucial in enhancing students' learning experiences. Students spoke at length about the qualities of and the manner in which they were drawn in by the vibrant colours and sophisticated quilting techniques (layering, piecing and machine sewing) that lent a three-dimensional quality to the depicted end-of-life scenes. We doubt that the same learning benefits could be obtained by using pictures of artwork in a book.

The results we obtained from this intervention may also be explained by recent research on mirror neurons, which neuroscientists newly perceive as the seat of empathy in the brain (e.g., Carr, Iacoboni, Dubeau, Mazziotta & Lenzi, 2003; Gallese, 2003). Mirror neurons are brain cells "specialized in understanding our existential condition and our involvement with others" (Iacoboni, 2008, p. 267) and facilitate the establishment of empathetic bonds between people. Freedberg and Gallese (2007) argue that artwork produces physiologic reactions as these mirror neurons facilitate "the direct experiential understanding of the intentional and emotional contents of images" (p. 202). They cite neuroimaging evidence that shows these empathetic responses to have "a precise and definable material basis in the brain" (p. 202). Similarly, Jeffers (2009) discusses "the mirror neuron system that can explain how students connect to and are connected by their interactions with objects of art, the artists producing them, and the classmates with whom they share a 'we-centered' space" (p. 11). This research suggests that empathetic engagement could be effectively triggered by observing works depicting scenes that elicit an empathetic response. Our findings therefore lend credence to these neuroesthetic arguments that effective learning is more likely to occur when powerful sensory experiences are triggered in the limbic system, the part of the brain that regulates emotional response (Hinton, Miyamoto & Della-Chiesa, 2008; Ingleton, 2002).

One caveat of our study is that students viewed original artwork in an art gallery; the immediacy of this experience arguably provides a greater impact than would viewing reproductions of the same artwork in a classroom. However, this disparity in impact could be overcome by displaying artwork on high-definition computer monitors or TV screens, thus enhancing its vividness and emotional force. Using visual art in this manner is both pedagogically advantageous and convenient because the images can be uploaded from scanned prints, digital pictures or searchable educational databases. Furthermore, instructors could design interventions around works representing specific medical conditions, patient populations or illness circumstances (Murray, 2000). Many websites also feature readily searchable databases containing downloadable annotated pictures. One well-known example is the Literature, Arts, and Medicine Database maintained by the Division of Educational Informatics at New York University School of Medicine (Holden, 2007). In addition, several artists have produced work on specific illnesses (Murray, 2000): Robert Pope's (1991) *Illness and healing* series of paintings famously chronicles his struggle with Hodgkin's disease, for example. Pope's work has been used in medical schools across Canada and the United States to teach students how to engage empathetically with cancer patients. In this way, the flexibility and focus afforded by reproduced artwork may in fact represent a pedagogical advantage over students' attendance at an independent gallery exhibit.

Others caveats include sampling self-selection, sample representativeness and sample size. Although self-selection is unavoidable in qualitative research, it is possible that this study involved participants with an above-average appreciation of the arts; students with a lesser appreciation might respond less successfully to the exercises.

A second concern is that our sample included four women and one man; our findings thus over-represent the experiences of women in regard to this intervention. However, we did not detect a gender difference in the data: the male student and female students reported similar appreciation of the artwork, and we observed them to be equally engaged in the role-playing exercises. A final issue is the small size of our sample. While having only five medical students take part in this pilot study proved ideal for gathering in-depth data about their experiences, our findings are obviously limited by their lack of generalizability to a larger population. Further research based on a larger, representative sample of medical students would help gauge more accurately the effectiveness of this intervention. These caveats aside, we want to emphasize that while this intervention involved medical students, it is by no means discipline specific. Further research on the intervention's applicability across a variety of disciplines would help establish protocols for adapting the intervention to serve the learning needs of students and health care providers in all disciplines.

Conclusion

Until recently, the issue of empathy training was hampered by "decades-old arguments in the literature voicing the concern that empathy interferes with scientific and medical objectivity" (Garden, 2007, p. 553). The consequences of dismissing empathy in medical education have been well documented: medical students learn to suppress their emotions and find it increasingly difficult to empathize with patients as their clinical training progresses (Beaudoin et al., 1998; Bellini, Baime & Shea, 2002; Newton et al., 2000; Sinclair, 1997; Wilkes, Milgrom & Hoffman, 2002). In his analysis of physicians' first-person accounts of their medical school experiences, Conrad (1988) concludes:

> Medical education emphasizes disease, technical procedures, and technological medicine, with scant attention to "caring" aspects of doctoring. Students struggle to learn medicine and to maintain a humanistic or patient-oriented perspective, but the social environment of medical training militates against humanistic doctoring. (p. 323)

Empathy's devaluation as a clinical skill means that training programs in empathy are often insufficiently supported, forcing students to rely on lectures, which are convenient but do not give students the opportunity to practice empathetic techniques (Henry-Tillman, Deloney, Savidge, Graham & Klimberg, 2002; Stepien & Baernstein,

2006). Shapiro (2008) notes that medical education still "does not include sufficiently thorough preparation to reflect on, be present with, and come to terms with [students'] fear and anxiety about being contaminated by patients' confusion, loss, vulnerability, helplessness, powerlessness, and suffering—and their own" (p. 5).

Our intervention addresses this paucity of training with an experiential and convenient protocol designed to encourage students in developing empathy skills early in their training. First- and second-year medical students participating in this study experienced empathetic responses to the circumstances of illness, death and dying depicted in the artwork they viewed under the guidance of an applied-arts facilitator. The peer-to-peer interactions and group session helped students share their views and experiences of empathy. The results suggest this intervention represents an important first step in prompting students to cultivate emotional self-awareness and empathetic responses to patients in end-of-life health care situations. The intervention also marks a point of departure for further cultivation of empathy skills, which, as Halpern (2001) notes, can only be refined over a lifetime of clinical work with self-education and self-awareness.

In conclusion, we suggest that empathy training would be even more beneficial if it also integrated learning about how social inequities mediate patients' experiences of illness (e.g., Link & Phelan, 1995; Wilkinson, 1997). Much of the literature on empathy training focuses almost exclusively on ways to improve clinical communication skills. However, as Garden (2007) notes, truly effective empathy needs to "extend beyond the individual relation to address socially determined inequities in health care" (p. 563). Similarly, Wear and Aultman (2005) recommend a more critical approach to teaching in medical settings that deepen "students' willingness to imagine what it is like to be someone who is suffering, and to work against oppressive social structures that sustain such suffering" (p. 1056). This expansion of empathy training would involve students in examining how illness impacts individuals differently depending on their economic status. In the case of our intervention, training would require the use of suitable artwork to illustrate how the poorest patients are at a higher risk of illness (Wilkinson, 1997) and the least likely to have access to adequate health services (Chappell & Penning, 2001; Denton, Prus & Walters, 2004; Nazroo, 2003). The intention would be to give students the opportunity to empathize with patients by understanding how disadvantageous socio-economic circumstances can contribute to their ill health.

NOTES

This article was originally published in *The International Journal of the Creative Arts in Interdisciplinary Practice*, IJCAIP, issue #10, November, 2011.

We would like to acknowledge Deidre Scherer for her exceptional skill in depicting palliative-care scenes through fabric art. We would also like to acknowledge the Greater Victoria Eldercare Foundation for supporting Embrace Aging Month in Victoria, BC, by arranging for this art exhibit to be shown at the University of Victoria. Funding was received from Canadian Institutes of Health Research (CIHR) New Emerging Team Grant ("Overcoming Barriers to Effective Communication in the Transition to Palliative/End of Life Care"). The New Emerging Team (NET) grants component of the Palliative and End-of-Life Care initiative is designed to build capacity and to promote the formation of new research teams or the growth of small existing teams. We received further support from the Centre on Aging, University of Victoria, and their Research Unit Infrastructure Grant from the Michael Smith Foundation for Health Research.

1 The scientific turn in medicine can be traced to the 1910 Flexner Report, which resulted in American and Canadian medical schools enacting higher training standards based on the principles of human physiology and biochemistry (Beck, 2004). The Flexner Report is credited with improving medical training, but it also diminished interest in the interpersonal component of medical practice (Hays & DiMatteo, 1984, p. 6).

2 See www.dscherer.com for sample images of some of the artwork viewed by medical students.

3 This conceptualization of empathy originates from German philosopher Robert Vischer's work on aesthetics. In 1873, he coined the term *Einfühlung* ("in-feeling" or "feeling-into") to capture the process by which human beings project feelings onto the natural world (Montag, Gallinat & Heinz, 2008). Theodor Lipps, a fellow philosopher, popularized the concept by using it to explain the human ability to imagine another's perspective. The term *Einfühlung* was translated to English in 1909 as "empathy" by famed British psychologist Edward Titchener in an effort to distinguish it from the then-popular notion of sympathy (Jahoda, 2005).

4 Phenomenographic and phenomenological research share similarities: both approaches are relational, experiential, content oriented and qualitative (Marton, 1986). However, phenomenography also differs substantively from phenomenology. The latter constitutes a philosophical method that seeks to capture a phenomenon's essence (Creswell, 2007). By contrast, phenomenographers adopt a more modest empirical orientation toward phenomena, seeking to articulate participants' reflections on experience as completely as possible (Marton & Booth, 1997).

REFERENCES

Anderson, R., & Schiedermayer, D. (2003, Jun). The Art of Medicine through the Humanities: an overview of a one-month humanities elective for fourth year students. *Medical Education, 37*(6), 560–562. http://dx.doi.org/10.1046/j.1365-2923.2003.01538.x Medline:12787380

Bardes, C.L., Gillers, D., & Herman, A.E. (2001, Dec). Learning to look: developing clinical observational skills at an art museum. *Medical Education, 35*(12), 1157–1161. http://dx.doi.org/10.1046/j.1365-2923.2001.01088.x Medline:11895244

Barnard, D. (1994, Aug). Making a place for the humanities in residency education. *Academic Medicine, 69*(8), 628–630. http://dx.doi.org/10.1097/00001888-199408000-00004 Medline:8054104

Beaudoin, C., Maheux, B., Côté, L., Des Marchais, J.E., Jean, P., & Berkson, L. (1998, Oct 6). Clinical teachers as humanistic caregivers and educators: perceptions of senior clerks and second-year residents. *Canadian Medical Association Journal, 159*(7), 765–769. Medline:9805021

Beck, A.H. (2004, May 5). STUDENTJAMA. The Flexner report and the standardization of American medical education. *Journal of the American Medical Association, 291*(17), 2139–2140. http://dx.doi.org/10.1001/jama.291.17.2139 Medline:15126445

Begley, A.M. (1996). Literature and poetry: Pleasure and practice. *International Journal of Nursing Practice*, *2*(4), 182–188. http://dx.doi.org/10.1111/j.1440-172X.1996.tb00050.x

Bellini, L.M., Baime, M., & Shea, J.A. (2002, Jun 19). Variation of mood and empathy during internship. *Journal of the American Medical Association*, *287*(23), 3143–3146. http://dx.doi.org/10.1001/jama.287.23.3143 Medline:12069680

Bereiter, C. (1992). Referent-centred and problem-centred knowledge: Elements of an educational epistemology. *Interchange*, *23*(4), 337–361. http://dx.doi.org/10.1007/BF01447280

Bereiter, C., & Scardamalia, M. (1996). Rethinking learning. In D.R. Olson & N. Torrance (Eds.), *The handbook of education and human development: New models of learning, teaching and schooling* (pp. 485–513). Cambridge, MA: Basil Blackwell.

Bleakley, A., Marshall, R., & Brömer, R. (2006, Winter). Toward an aesthetic medicine: developing a core medical humanities undergraduate curriculum. *Journal of Medical Humanities*, *27*(4), 197–213. http://dx.doi.org/10.1007/s10912-006-9018-5 Medline:17096192

Blomqvist, L., Pitkälä, K., & Routasalo, P. (2007, Mar–Apr). Images of loneliness: using art as an educational method in professional training. *Journal of Continuing Education in Nursing*, *38*(2), 89–93. Medline:17402381

Bolton, G.M. (1984). *Drama as education: An argument for placing drama at the centre of the curriculum*. London: Longman.

Booth, D. (2003). Towards an understanding of theatre for education. In K. Gallagher & D. Booth (Eds.), *How theatre educates: Convergences and counterpoints with artists, scholars, and advocates* (pp. 15–22). Toronto, ON: University of Toronto Press.

Brett-MacLean, P., & Yiu, V. (2006). Exploring the art of medicine. *Canadian Creative Arts in Health, Training and Education eNews/journal*, *3*, 6–7.

Butow, P.N., Maclean, M., Dunn, S.M., Tattersall, M.H.N., & Boyer, M.J. (1997, Sep). The dynamics of change: cancer patients' preferences for information, involvement and support. *Annals of Oncology*, *8*(9), 857–863. http://dx.doi.org/10.1023/A:1008284006045 Medline:9358935

Calman, K. (2001). A study of storytelling, humour and learning in medicine. *Clinical Medicine*, *1*(3), 227–229. Medline:11446621

Calman, K., & Downie, R. (1996, Jun 1). Why arts courses for medical curricula. *Lancet*, *347*(9014), 1499–1500. http://dx.doi.org/10.1016/S0140-6736(96)90665-0 Medline:8684096

Carr, L., Iacoboni, M., Dubeau, M.C., Mazziotta, J.C., & Lenzi, G.L. (2003, Apr 29). Neural mechanisms of empathy in humans: a relay from neural systems for imitation to limbic areas. *Proceedings of the National Academy of Sciences of the United States of America*, *100*(9), 5497–5502. http://dx.doi.org/10.1073/pnas.0935845100 Medline:12682281

Castledine, G. (1998, Apr 23). Link between the arts and the experience of nursing. *British Journal of Nursing (Mark Allen Publishing)*, *7*(8), 493. Medline:9668770

Chappell, N.L., & Penning, M.J. (2001). Sociology of aging in Canada: Issues for the millennium. *Canadian Journal on Aging*, *20*(S1 suppl), 82–110. http://dx.doi.org/10.1017/S0714980800015233

Charon, R. (2001, Oct 17). The patient–physician relationship. Narrative medicine: a model for empathy, reflection, profession, and trust. *Journal of the American Medical Association*, *286*(15), 1897–1902. http://dx.doi.org/10.1001/jama.286.15.1897 Medline:11597295

Cohen, L.M. (2001). Review of Scherer, D. (1998). Deidre Scherer: Work in fabric and thread. Concord, CA: C & T Publishing. *Psychosomatics*, *42*(4), 374. http://dx.doi.org/10.1176/appi.psy.42.4.374

Conrad, P. (1988, Dec). Learning to doctor: reflections on recent accounts of the medical school years. *Journal of Health and Social Behavior*, *29*(4), 323–332. http://dx.doi.org/10.2307/2136866 Medline:3253323

Creswell, J.W. (2007). *Qualitative inquiry and research design: Choosing among five traditions* (2nd ed.). Thousand Oaks, CA: Sage.

DasGupta, S., & Charon, R. (2004, Apr). Personal illness narratives: using reflective writing to teach empathy. *Academic Medicine, 79*(4), 351–356. http://dx.doi.org/10.1097/00001888-200404000-00013 Medline:15044169

Deeney, P., Johnson, A., Boore, J., Leyden, C., & McCaughan, E. (2001). Drama as an experiential technique in learning how to cope with dying patients and their families. *Teaching in Higher Education, 6*(1), 99–112.

Deloney, L.A., & Graham, C.J. (2003, Fall). *Wit*: using drama to teach first-year medical students about empathy and compassion. *Teaching and Learning in Medicine, 15*(4), 247–251. http://dx.doi.org/10.1207/S15328015TLM1504_06 Medline:14612257

Denton, M., Prus, S., & Walters, V. (2004, Jun). Gender differences in health: a Canadian study of the psychosocial, structural and behavioural determinants of health. *Social Science & Medicine, 58*(12), 2585–2600. http://dx.doi.org/10.1016/j.socscimed.2003.09.008 Medline:15081207

DeVito, J.A. (1999). *Messages: Building interpersonal communication skills*. New York: Addison-Wesley Educational Publishers, Inc.

Dickinson, G.E. (2007, Sep). End-of-life and palliative care issues in medical and nursing schools in the United States. *Death Studies, 31*(8), 713–726. http://dx.doi.org/10.1080/07481180701490602 Medline:17853525

Dolev, J.C., Friedlaender, L.K., & Braverman, I.M. (2001, Sep 5). Use of fine art to enhance visual diagnostic skills. *Journal of the American Medical Association, 286*(9), 1020–1021. http://dx.doi.org/10.1001/jama.286.9.1020 Medline:11559280

Ekebergh, M., Lepp, M., & Dahlberg, K. (2004, Nov). Reflective learning with drama in nursing education—a Swedish attempt to overcome the theory praxis gap. *Nurse Education Today, 24*(8), 622–628. http://dx.doi.org/10.1016/j.nedt.2004.07.011 Medline:15519445

Elizur, A., & Rosenheim, E. (1982, Sep). Empathy and attitudes among medical students: the effects of group experience. *Journal of Medical Education, 57*(9), 675–683. Medline:7202049

Freedberg, D., & Gallese, V. (2007, May). Motion, emotion and empathy in esthetic experience. *Trends in Cognitive Sciences, 11*(5), 197–203. http://dx.doi.org/10.1016/j.tics.2007.02.003 Medline:17347026

Gallese, V. (2003, Jul–Aug). The roots of empathy: the shared manifold hypothesis and the neural basis of intersubjectivity. *Psychopathology, 36*(4), 171–180. http://dx.doi.org/10.1159/000072786 Medline:14504450

Garden, R. (2007). The problem of empathy: Medicine and the humanities. *New Literary History, 38*(3), 551–567. http://dx.doi.org/10.1353/nlh.2007.0037

Halpern, J. (2001). *From detached concern to empathy: Humanizing medical practice*. New York: Oxford University Press.

Halpern, J. (2003, Aug). What is clinical empathy? *Journal of General Internal Medicine, 18*(8), 670–674. http://dx.doi.org/10.1046/j.1525-1497.2003.21017.x Medline:12911651

Hays, R., & DiMatteo, M.R. (1984). Toward a more therapeutic physician–patient relationship. In S. Duck (Ed.), *Personal relationships 5: Repairing personal relationships* (pp. 1–20). London: Academic Press.

Henry-Tillman, R., Deloney, L.A., Savidge, M., Graham, C.J., & Klimberg, V.S. (2002, Jun). The medical student as patient navigator as an approach to teaching empathy. *American Journal of Surgery, 183*(6), 659–662. http://dx.doi.org/10.1016/S0002-9610(02)00867-X Medline:12095596

Hinton, C., Miyamoto, K., & Della-Chiesa, B. (2008). Brain research, learning and emotions: Implications for education research, policy and practice. *European Journal of Education, 43*(1), 87–103. http://dx.doi.org/10.1111/j.1465-3435.2007.00336.x

Hoffman, S.B., Brand, F.R., Beatty, P.G., & Hamill, L.A. (1985, Dec). Geriatrix: a role-playing game. *Gerontologist, 25*(6), 568–572. http://dx.doi.org/10.1093/geront/25.6.568 Medline:4085868

Hojat, M., Gonnella, J.S., Nasca, T.J., Mangione, S., Vergare, M., & Magee, M. (2002, Sep). Physician empathy: definition, components, measurement, and relationship to gender and specialty. *American Journal of Psychiatry, 159*(9), 1563–1569. http://dx.doi.org/10.1176/appi.ajp.159.9.1563 Medline:12202278

Holden, C. (2007). Random samples. NETWATCH: Ill literacy. *Science, 316*(5832), 1675d. http://dx.doi.org/10.1126/science.316.5832.1675d

Iacoboni, M. (2008). *Mirroring people: The new science of how we connect with others.* New York: Farrar, Straus & Giroux.

Ingleton, C. (2002). Emotion in learning—a neglected dynamic. *Research and Development in Higher Education, 22,* 86–99.

Jahoda, G. (2005, Spring). Theodor Lipps and the shift from "sympathy" to "empathy." *Journal of the History of the Behavioral Sciences, 41*(2), 151–163. http://dx.doi.org/10.1002/jhbs.20080 Medline:15812816

Jeffers, C.S. (2009). On empathy: The mirror neuron system and art education. *International Journal of Education & the Arts,* 10(15). Retrieved August 10, 2010 from http://www.ijea.org/v10n15/.

Johansson, B., Marton, F., & Svensson, L. (1985). An approach to describing learning as change between qualitatively different conceptions. In L. West & A. Pines (Eds.), *Cognitive structure and conceptual change* (pp. 233–258). Orlando, FL: Academic Press.

Kidd, M.G., & Connor, J.T.H. (2008, Mar). Striving to do good things: teaching humanities in Canadian medical schools. *Journal of Medical Humanities, 29*(1), 45–54. http://dx.doi.org/10.1007/s10912-007-9049-6 Medline:18058208

Kirk, T.W. (2011). The meaning, limitations and possibilities of making palliative care a public health priority by declaring it a human right. *Public Health Ethics, 4*(1), 84–92. http://dx.doi.org/10.1093/phe/phr002

Lancaster, T., Hart, R., & Gardner, S. (2002, Nov). Literature and medicine: evaluating a special study module using the nominal group technique. *Medical Education, 36*(11), 1071–1076. http://dx.doi.org/10.1046/j.1365-2923.2002.01325.x Medline:12406268

Larson, E.B., & Yao, X. (2005, Mar 2). Clinical empathy as emotional labor in the patient–physician relationship. *Journal of the American Medical Association, 293*(9), 1100–1106. http://dx.doi.org/10.1001/jama.293.9.1100 Medline:15741532

Lazarus, P.A., & Rosslyn, F.M. (2003, Jun). The Arts in Medicine: setting up and evaluating a new special study module at Leicester Warwick Medical School. *Medical Education, 37*(6), 553–559. http://dx.doi.org/10.1046/j.1365-2923.2003.01537.x Medline:12787379

Lewis, P., & Johnson, D.R. (2000). *Current approaches in drama therapy.* Springfield, IL: Charles C. Thomas.

Link, B.G., & Phelan, J. (1995). Social conditions as fundamental causes of disease. *Journal of Health and Social Behavior, 35*(Spec No), 80–94. http://dx.doi.org/10.2307/2626958 Medline:7560851

Marton, F. (1986). Phenomenography: A research approach investigating different understandings of reality. *Journal of Thought, 21*(2), 28–49.

Marton, F. (1988). Phenomenography: Exploring different conceptions of reality. In D.M. Fetterman (Ed.), *Qualitative approaches to evaluation in education: The silent scientific revolution* (pp. 176–205). New York: Praeger.

Marton, F., & Booth, S. (1997). *Learning and awareness.* Mahwah, NJ: Lawerence Erlbaum Associates.

Marton, F., & Pong, W. (2005). On the unit of description in phenomenography. *Higher Education Research & Development, 24*(4), 335–348. http://dx.doi.org/10.1080/07294360500284706

McManus, I.C. (1995, Oct 28). Humanity and the medical humanities. *Lancet, 346*(8983), 1143–1145. http://dx.doi.org/10.1016/S0140-6736(95)91806-X Medline:7475609

Meryn, S. (1998, Jun 27). Improving doctor–patient communication. Not an option, but a necessity. *British Medical Journal, 316*(7149), 1922–1930. http://dx.doi.org/10.1136/bmj.316.7149.1922 Medline:9641926

Montag, C., Gallinat, J., & Heinz, A. (2008, Oct). Theodor Lipps and the concept of empathy: 1851–1914. *American Journal of Psychiatry, 165*(10), 1261. http://dx.doi.org/10.1176/appi.ajp.2008.07081283 Medline:18829882

Morse, J.M., Bottorff, J., Anderson, G., O'Brien, B., & Solberg, S. (1992, Jul). Beyond empathy: expanding expressions of caring. *Journal of Advanced Nursing, 17*(7), 809–821. http://dx.doi.org/10.1111/j.1365-2648.1992.tb02002.x Medline:1644977

Moyle, W., Barnard, A., & Turner, C. (1995, May). The humanities and nursing: using popular literature as a means of understanding human experience. *Journal of Advanced Nursing, 21*(5), 960–964. http://dx.doi.org/10.1046/j.1365-2648.1995.21050960.x Medline:7602005

Murray, T.J. (2000, Jan 4). Personal time: the patient's experience. *Annals of Internal Medicine, 132*(1), 58–62. http://dx.doi.org/10.7326/0003-4819-132-1-200001040-00010 Medline:10627253

Nazroo, J.Y. (2003, Feb). The structuring of ethnic inequalities in health: economic position, racial discrimination, and racism. *American Journal of Public Health, 93*(2), 277–284. http://dx.doi.org/10.2105/AJPH.93.2.277 Medline:12554585

Newton, B.W., Savidge, M.A., Barber, L., et al. (2000, Dec). Differences in medical students' empathy. *Academic Medicine, 75*(12), 1215. http://dx.doi.org/10.1097/0000 1888-200012000-00020 Medline:11112725

Nordgren, L., & Olsson, H. (2004, Feb). Palliative care in a coronary care unit: a qualitative study of physicians' and nurses' perceptions. *Journal of Clinical Nursing, 13*(2), 185–193. http://dx.doi.org/10.1111/j.1365-2702.2004.00816.x Medline: 14723670

Northcott, H.C., & Wilson, D.M. (2008). *Dying and death in Canada.* Peterborough, ON: Broadview Press.

Ousager, J., & Johannessen, H. (2010, Jun). Humanities in undergraduate medical education: a literature review. *Academic Medicine, 85*(6), 988–998. http://dx.doi.org/ 10.1097/ACM.0b013e3181dd226b Medline:20505399

Piette, J.D., Heisler, M., Krein, S., & Kerr, E.A. (2005, Aug 8–22). The role of patient-physician trust in moderating medication nonadherence due to cost pressures. *Archives of Internal Medicine, 165*(15), 1749–1755. http://dx.doi.org/10.1001/archinte.165.15. 1749 Medline:16087823

Pope, R. (1991). *Illness and healing: Images of cancer.* Hantsport, NS: Lancelot Press.

Price, A.M. (2004, May–Jun). Intensive care nurses' experiences of assessing and dealing with patients' psychological needs. *Nursing in Critical Care, 9*(3), 134–142. http://dx.doi. org/10.1111/j.1362-1017.2004.00055.x Medline:15152755

Richardson, J.T. (1999). The concepts and methods of phenomenographic research. *Review of Educational Research, 69*(1), 53–82. http://dx.doi.org/10.3102/00346543069 001053

Risse, G.B. (1992, Apr). Literature and medicine. *Western Journal of Medicine, 156*(4), 431. Medline:1574896

Ross, C.W. (1978, Jan–Feb). Nurses' personal death concerns and responses to dying-patient statements. *Nursing Research, 27*(1), 64–68. http://dx.doi.org/10.1097/00006199-19780 1000-00030 Medline:244890

Roter, D.L., Stewart, M., Putnam, S.M., Lipkin, M., Jr., Stiles, W., & Inui, T.S. (1997, Jan 22–29). Communication patterns of primary care physicians. *Journal of the American Medical Association, 277*(4), 350–356. http://dx.doi.org/10.1001/jama.1997.03540280088045 Medline:9002500

Scherer, D. (1998). *Deidre Scherer: Work in fabric and thread.* Concord, CA: C & T Publishing.

Shapiro, J. (2008). Walking a mile in their patients' shoes: empathy and othering in medical students' education. *Philosophy, Ethics, and Humanities in Medicine; PEHM, 3,* 10. http://dx.doi.org/10.1186/1747-5341-3-10 Medline:18336719

Shapiro, J., & Hunt, L. (2003, Oct). All the world's a stage: the use of theatrical performance in medical education. *Medical Education, 37*(10), 922–927. http://dx.doi. org/10.1046/j.1365-2923.2003.01634.x Medline:12974849

Sinclair, S. (1997). *Making doctors: An institutional apprenticeship.* Oxford, UK: Berg.

Skelton, J.R., Macleod, J.A.A., & Thomas, C.P. (2000, Dec 9). Teaching literature and medicine to medical students, part II: why literature and medicine? *Lancet, 356*(9246), 2001–2003. http://dx.doi.org/10.1016/S0140-6736(00)03318-3 Medline:11130538

Smith, B.H. (1998, Jun). Literature in our medical schools. *British Journal of General Practice, 48*(431), 1337–1340. Medline:9747554

Spencer, L., Ritchie, J., & O'Connor, W. (2003). Focus groups. In J. Ritchie & J. Lewis (Eds.), *Qualitative research practice: A guide for social science students and researchers* (pp. 170–198). London: Sage.

Starr, P. (1982). *The social transformation of American medicine.* New York: Basic Books.

Stepien, K.A., & Baernstein, A. (2006, May). Educating for empathy. A review. *Journal of General Internal Medicine, 21*(5), 524–530. http://dx.doi.org/10.1111/j.1525-1497.2006.00443.x Medline:16704404

Stowe, A.C., & Igo, L.C. (1996, Sep–Oct). Learning from literature: novels, plays, short stories, and poems in nursing education. *Nurse Educator, 21*(5), 16–19. http://dx.doi.org/10.1097/00006223-199609000-00008 Medline:8936177

Suchman, A.L., Markakis, K., Beckman, H.B., & Frankel, R. (1997, Feb 26). A model of empathic communication in the medical interview. *Journal of the American Medical Association, 277*(8), 678–682. http://dx.doi.org/10.1001/jama.1997.03540320082047 Medline:9039890

Trigwell, K.Rust, C. (Ed.) (2000). Phenomenography: Variation and discernment. In C. Rust (Ed.), *Improving student learning. Proceedings of the 1999 7th International Symposium* (pp. 75–85). Oxford, UK: Oxford Centre for Staff and Learning Development.

Wasylko, Y., & Stickley, T. (2003, Aug). Theatre and pedagogy: using drama in mental health nurse education. *Nurse Education Today, 23*(6), 443–448. http://dx.doi.org/10.1016/S0260-6917(03)00046-7 Medline:12900193

Wear, D., & Aultman, J.M. (2005, Oct). The limits of narrative: medical student resistance to confronting inequality and oppression in literature and beyond. *Medical Education, 39*(10), 1056–1065. http://dx.doi.org/10.1111/j.1365-2929.2005.02270.x Medline:16178833

Welch, T.R., & Welch, M. (2008, Aug). Dramatic insights: a report of the effects of a dramatic production on the learning of student nurses during their mental health course component. *International Journal of Mental Health Nursing, 17*(4), 261–269. http://dx.doi.org/10.1111/j.1447-0349.2008.00542.x Medline:18666909

Wikström, B.-M. (2001, Feb). Work of art dialogues: an educational technique by which students discover personal knowledge of empathy. *International Journal of Nursing Practice, 7*(1), 24–29. http://dx.doi.org/10.1046/j.1440-172x.2001.00248.x Medline: 11811344

Wikström, B.-M. (2003, Jan–Feb). A picture of a work of art as an empathy teaching strategy in nurse education complementary to theoretical knowledge. *Journal of Professional Nursing, 19*(1), 49–54. http://dx.doi.org/10.1053/jpnu.2003.5 Medline:12649819

Wilkes, M., Milgrom, E., & Hoffman, J.R. (2002, Jun). Towards more empathic medical students: a medical student hospitalization experience. *Medical Education, 36*(6), 528–533. http://dx.doi.org/10.1046/j.1365-2923.2002.01230.x Medline:12047666

Wilkinson, R.G. (1997). *Unhealthy societies: The afflictions of inequality.* London: Routledge.

Wolf, T.M., Balson, P.M., Faucett, J.M., & Randall, H.M. (1989, Jan). A retrospective study of attitude change during medical education. *Medical Education, 23*(1), 19–23. http://dx.doi.org/10.1111/j.1365-2923.1989.tb00807.x Medline:2927336

World Health Organization. (2007). *Palliative Care (Cancer Control: Knowledge into Action: WHO Guide for Effective Programmes; Module 5).* Geneva, Switzerland: World Health Organization.

Correspondence: André Smith, Department of Sociology, University of Victoria, Cor A333, 3800 Finnerty Road, Victoria, BC V8W 3P5. E-mail: apsmith@uvic.ca

2

Remember Me for Birds

An Ethnodrama about Aging, Mental Health and Autonomy

Cheryl L. McLean

The mission of art is to bring out the unfamiliar from the most familiar.

—Khalil Gibran (1966)

In this article I will share my process as I researched and wrote a performance that I developed into an ethnodrama about aging, mental health and autonomy, based on true stories.

Background

While studying and doing graduate research at Concordia University, I worked for two years as a drama therapist associated with an Over-60 mental-health program in Montreal. Working with older people living in low-income residential homes, I used drama methods in group therapy. All of my clients were Jewish and among them were Holocaust survivors. During that time I witnessed first-hand that lack of autonomy contributed to stress and depression for several of my older clients. When informally surveyed, these older men and women indicated lack of autonomy was the issue that concerned them most about resident life.

By lack of autonomy, or compromised independence, I mean the inability to make decisions about one's life and restrictions around personal freedoms (what to eat, when to eat, access to personal money, transportation services, issues around relocation). I also found that, on the whole, there were few resources available for older people for preventive therapies that could help address their mental-health issues.

While studying in Montreal, I worked as an actor on several projects with Dr. Muriel Gold, a seasoned theatre professional and formerly the artistic director of the Saidye Bronfman Theatre. She was also a university acting teacher who was familiar with drama with special populations. Muriel introduced me to Stanislavski acting methods (realism) and self-exploration as a basis for character development where "preparation exercises aim to stimulate participants to look inward, to explore their own inner resources and narratives in order to build experiences from which they can develop believable characters" (Gold, 2000, p. 6).

The use of narrative in health has made significant inroads, particularly in narrative medicine, an approach pioneered by Charon (2008), who has long advocated the use of narrative in medical education to honour stories of illness.

Denzin (2003) has established the connections between research inquiry, writing, narrative and performance ethnography. Denzin explains performance is an act of intervention, a method of resistance, a form of criticism, a way of revealing agency: "performance becomes public pedagogy when it uses the aesthetic, the performative, to foreground the intersection of politics, institutional sites and embodied experience" (Denzin, 2003, p. 9).

Ethnodrama, a qualitative approach considered a form of ethnographic theatre, is an emerging genre, an embodied and multisensory form of research that has much to offer both education and health care. Saldaña (2011) offers further insight with a definition of ethnodrama:

> An ethnodrama ... is a written play script consisting of dramatized, significant selections of narrative collected from interview transcripts, participant observation, field notes, journal entries, personal memories/experiences and/or print and media artifacts such as diaries, blogs, e-mail correspondence, television broadcasts, newspaper articles, court proceedings and historical documents. ... Simply put, this is dramatizing the data.[1] (p. 13)

If there is one overarching feature that distinguishes ethnodrama as a research-based art form from fictional dramatic plays, it is that the performance is about true stories. Saldaña (2011) explains that ethnotheatre

> employs the traditional craft and artistic techniques of theatre or media production to mount for an audience a live or mediated performance event of research participants' experiences and/or the researcher's interpretations of data ... the goal is to investigate a particular facet of the human condition for purposes of adapting those observations and insights into a performance medium. This investigation is preparatory fieldwork for theatrical production work. (p. 12)

Saldaña stresses the importance of aesthetic integrity and theatrical quality for these rich and multi-faceted performances. Ethnodrama is researched and constructed based on reality, but it should do more than present facts and inform. The ethnodrama script and performance must be compelling enough to hold and entertain an audience:

> With ethnographic performance ... comes the responsibility to create an entertainingly informative experience for an audience, one that is aesthetically sound, intellectually rich, and emotionally evocative. Ethnotheatre reveals a living culture through its character-participants and, if successful, the audience learns about their world and what it's like to live in it. (Saldaña, 2005, p. 14)

These are performances that can foster empathy and understanding by critically reflecting real-life experience.

Denzin (2003) explains:

> A performative discourse simultaneously writes and criticizes performances. In showing how people enact cultural meanings in their daily lives, such a discourse focuses on how these meanings and performances shape experiences of injustice, prejudice and stereotyping. (p. xi)

Drawing on my writing, acting and therapeutic experience and considering the challenges and goals of the research, I believed the best way to foster empathy and raise awareness about aging, mental health and autonomy was to write and act in a solo performance based on research and client stories. The performance would be staged for health care workers and those who worked in gerontology. Muriel Gold agreed to direct the performance and offered invaluable feedback during the creative process.

Process

Early in the research process, I immersed myself in tactile fact-gathering that started with my creating a floor collage. The collage began as a few newspaper articles and photographs and developed over time to

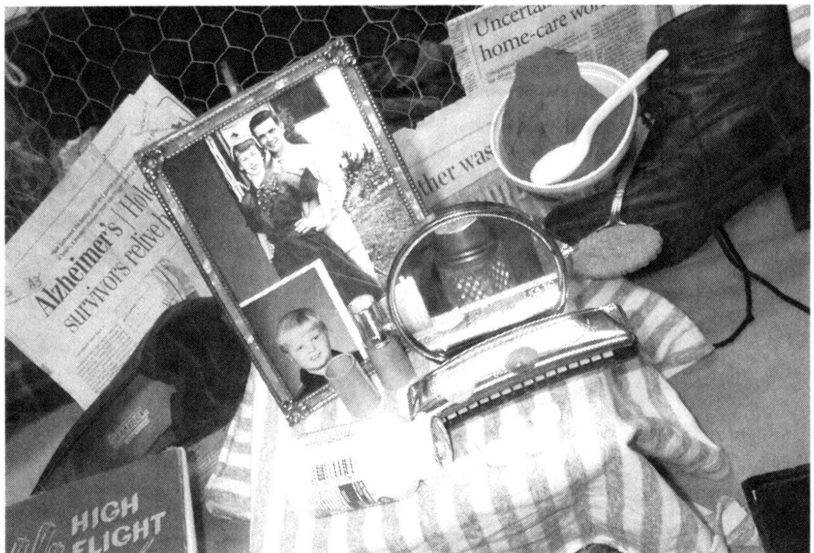

Figure 2.1 Process/collage objects set in working installation; photo by Constance Balsano

include client photos; line drawings of clients; client art and stories; case studies, transcripts and videotapes; ditties and songs about growing old; and found objects from the dining room (such as resident dinner menus, spoons, bowls and salt and pepper shakers).

This collage became my creative centre, a place for tactile multidimensional construction where I distilled and assimilated materials identifying issues of importance, among them transportation, food, support in crisis, diagnostic labeling, effects of past traumas, environmental triggering and relocations. Early in the process I used the collage to identify common themes, which I indicated in bold lettering across articles and photographs. I would at times contrast one issue with another, historical accounts with newspaper articles, seeking patterns in events past and present. Some of the found objects from the collage eventually became part of the set or were used as props during the performance. The spoon, for example, was one object particularly imbued with metaphor in this piece.

I sought to learn as much about my clients as possible, compiling detailed field notes, conducting one-on-one interviews, recording oral histories, taping selected therapy sessions, reading topical community-news stories, attending team meetings, talking with social workers and consulting journals of gerontology. I immersed myself physically within the context of my clients' environment, participating fully in resident life. I conducted interviews in one-room apartments, got to know the social workers, the staff and the building superintendent, attended social gatherings, shared in music performances and enjoyed lively conversations on park benches. The older people in the resident community shared their stories through participating in interviews and oral histories and when they engaged in story-making during our drama-therapy sessions, as well as when creating visual art and poetry. They were aware they would be the inspiration for a performance and offered their stories willingly to help others. I used the research information I gathered, much of it from working directly in the field, in my monologues, which made up the ethnodrama script about real-life issues affecting autonomy and mental health.

> Sometimes, in the telling, you may feel the past lives and present begins
> and yet no one has left this dining room.
> Inside/ soup bowls empty
> and yet, outside ... is still the long, long wait
> for change.
> But the voices tell us all is not lost,
> remembering is a beginning,
> like soup ... we are what we prepare
> and we have within our hands the bowl
> that could provide well for us all
> if we hold on to the spoon very carefully. (McLean, 2005, p. 16)

The monologues for *Remember me for birds* were constructed to lend voice to older people's issues and included local stories in the context of the resident environment contrasted with events shaped by personal histories. To protect individuals' identities, I did not use actual names, nor did I specify locations. In some cases compilation characters were used to reflect experiences from multiple sources. From the play notes:

> Caught in the fence, as if blown by wind, scraps of the local newspaper, the headlines visible, stories of elder abuse, ageism. On a small stool a telephone, the receiver off the hook, an empty pill bottle, a nurse's cap (circa 1964), a black and white photograph of a young man and woman dressed in the style of the 50s. There is a small table and a chair, on the table, a bowl and spoon, a set of salt and pepper shakers, a coffee mug. Downstage left a sheet with a pillow to indicate a small bed. (McLean, 2005, p. 15)

"Eddie" was a character based on a client, aged 78, who was new to the resident home. I had learned he had been very depressed since arriving at the facility several months previous to our first meeting. Eddie's monologue was constructed based on research from an oral history I gathered at the residence from four two-hour, one-on-one interview sessions that took place in his apartment. Eddie willingly provided written permission to use his story for the purposes of the performance. I tape-recorded and transcribed the sessions and took extensive notes. Later, I edited the transcripts and identified the main themes and issues that emerged. Many centred on issues of autonomy, such as concerns about transportation and particularly Eddie's regrets about being unable to drive.

I listened many times to Eddie's tape-recorded voice while I wrote the script, paying close attention to his voice changes and pauses, particularly during times that moved him most deeply. As an actor, I began to read the transcript carefully to embody the feelings behind Eddie's words, as well as noting the silences and nuances such as long pauses, throat clearing, breaths. Many of these revealing vocal characteristics were eventually incorporated into the performance itself.

> EDDIE:
>
> Before Frank died, he says to me, Eddie, I think you otta' see a psychiatrist, you are just not yourself, Eddie, you're getting forgetful Eddie, you need to talk to somebody, see a psychiatrist, Eddie ... and he was my brother, so ... I went. So there I was sittin' across from the psychiatrist, like I'm sittin' across from you, and the psychiatrist looks at me and he says ... how many sides does a pencil have? A pencil? (pause) (Eddie turns a "pencil" in his hand) Look, I had to remind the doctor three times what my name was. You tell me who has the bad memory?
>
> Doctors, hospitals it's my life these days ... they think I might have lung cancer, they think I've got a few spots, and I need to go the hospital to have some tests so I ask the girl here, who do I call to get a ride and she gives me the name of this guy from transportation services, and I call him and I say, look ... can you give me a ride to the hospital? (coughs, takes a breath) I have to get some tests, I have an appointment with the doctor, and he says yeah ... he'll come and get me, he's got a couple of people to pick up before me and he tells me I should go down to the lobby and he will be out in the parking lot. So I get ready, get my walker, go down the hall, down the elevator and out into the lobby and I wait. (Eddie is seen waiting with his walker, waiting, checking his watch ... the wait is just long enough for the audience to experience some impatience) I wait two hours for him to pick me up and he doesn't show up! (angry)
>
> Yeah ... I always had my cars. I could take off when I wanted, I used to pick up, I used to do. I never said no. (pause) Without my car I feel like I'm stuck here sitting like an idiot! And I never thought this would be the end of the road. (McLean, 2005, pp. 19–20)

Eddie projects his truth, and his story is representative of events at the residence and lived experience. He recalls his brother, "Frank," whom he misses dearly (he had died a few years earlier), and the concerns Frank had about his memory. Eddie expresses his feelings about visiting the psychiatrist and how he felt when his name was forgotten. He demonstrates the challenges he experienced trying to get a ride to the hospital to have tests to determine whether he had lung cancer. The waiting he experiences illustrates a systemic issue, that of unreliable transportation services. He also expresses his regrets about being unable to drive. Eddie's story dramatically embodies the many circumstances—both personal and environmental—that have contributed to his lack of autonomy and shows how these life stressors, one upon the other, compromised his mental health.

I also included survivors in the performance as their stories were of critical importance to individuals in the community and to the health workers who cared for them. Newspaper articles at the time were reporting that some aged survivors living in institutions continued to struggle with memories of the past.

"Dora" was a compilation character based on several Holocaust survivors I met and worked with over my two years as a therapist in Montreal. Historical accounts were also included in this scene. The performance demonstrated how the traumatic experiences of the Holocaust shaped Dora's behaviour in the context of resident life. She explains why she will not let anyone answer her door (a situation that can arise when nurses or social workers want to enter an apartment to assist) and why she screams when the "elevator" doors close (because she recalls being thrown into a cattle car for transport to the concentration camp). In this speech, history and past suffering are critically juxtaposed against current events, one situation mirroring the other. Behaviour that may be labeled as paranoid is embodied for the audience and presented through Dora's story in a revealing new context.

DORA:

Stealing ... thieves! They call me on the phone every day. They say, I want to help you clean your carpets. I want to help you fix your windows. I read in the newspaper they say, they are janitors or they are cleaning your carpets, they knock on your door, come into your house, poison your food, give you drugs, you pass out and they steal everything! Your jewelry, money! I never open the door to anyone. Lies! They want to send me to the hospital. Why? Why they want to send me to the hospital? I don't need any help! I am not sick. I saw the doctor and he said, Dora you gonna' live to be a hundred. The social worker she very nice. She say everything is good. Why they think I need help? I am very strong (pumps arm up and down) See ... I do exercises, up and down. I fix my own window (shows fixing window), I clean tub (shows cleaning the tub). I make soup. I ... make ... soup ... (pause, she reflects back) I make one bowl of soup, little bit garlic, salt, water. One bowl of soup feed twenty children. Children! Grown up today with children of their own. Working people. Alive!

They say, Dora, you calm down. You going crazy. They're going to send you to the hospital Dora, try to forget. Go on with your life. Take your pill. I say, why do

> you think I scream when I use the elevator here? Why do you think I scream? They threw us into cattle cars for six days without bread! They closed the doors, We could not breathe! (McLean, 2005, pp. 21–22)
>
> ...
>
> I am an old woman, but, I am alive.
> and I remember well.
> I wish that you will have a long life too.
> And that I will remember for you.
> So that, you will never suffer. (McLean, 2005, pp. 23)

This project evolved over several development stages. Initially I created four monologues representing clients, one man and three women. In the second phase of script development, over an additional year's time, scenes were added, as well as personal narratives, poems, video and audio to link and juxtapose ideas from past and present and to explain characters' personal connections to issues around themes of aging, autonomy and survival.

In the next speech, once again identifying issues around aging and autonomy and building on the survival theme, I reflected on my own grandfather's life, his past and his war experiences. At 17 years old, my grandfather left the little southern Ontario town of Leamington, "where people sold peaches and tomatoes at little road side stands," to

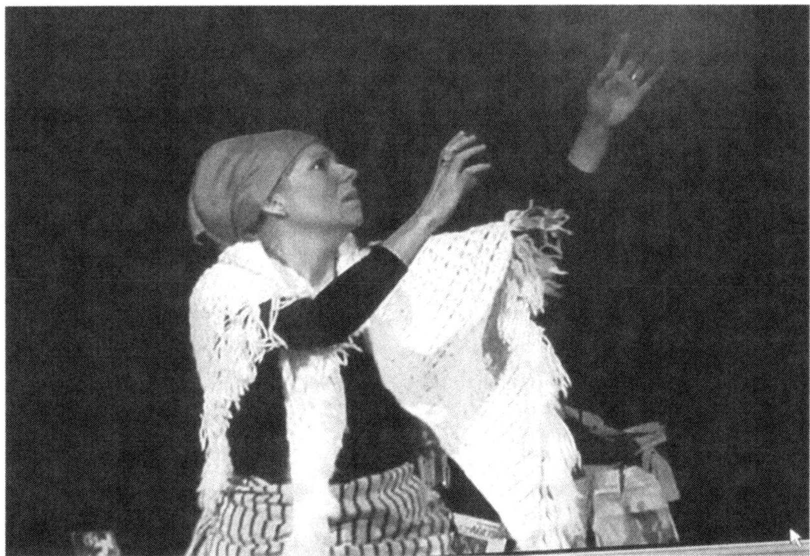

Figure 2.2 Cheryl McLean as "Dora" from the film version of the ethnodrama *Remember me for birds,* filmed by Aimee Edgcumbe

head for the battlefields of Europe to fight with the Canadian troops in the trenches at the Somme and Vimy Ridge. As I constructed this piece I found myself asking: What is autonomy? What does it mean to be free? Did my grandfather have any choice about what would become of him as a soldier in war, whether he would survive or die on the battlefield? My grandfather believed he was fighting for freedom. As a result of the war, the forces involved had suffered over 9 million deaths. My grandfather survived, but the war left lasting effects.

> MCLEAN:
> I remember / we would drive south to visit my grandfather,
> to the little retirement town of Leamington, Ontario,
> where people sold peaches and tomatoes at little road side stands,
> and lived in small white houses,
> like my grandfather's, where we would see him, sitting on the front porch
> reading the news
> and smoking one of his many cigars.
> My grandfather had a chronic cough
> not from the cigars he smoked,
> but from the poison gas ... he inhaled,
> in the trenches, during the First World War.
> He used to start coughing, and couldn't stop,
> his face would turn purple,
> And I would be afraid he was going to die.
> I could hear him in the bathroom gasping and wheezing.
> He never talked about the war.
> But I was a kid and I was curious and one day I asked him
> Grandpa did you ever kill anybody in the war?
> and he told me (grandpa's voice) It's too terrible to talk about.
> But one day he gathered us all 'round,
> And he brought out his war medals,
> in a small glass case (shows holding the case, picks up the medal)
> And it was the only time / I saw him / smile about the war.
> We wondered if the breast cancer he got was caused by the gas
> it eventually spread to his spine and killed him.
> I remember / he told me,
> (grandfather's voice) You know when I was a boy,
> I walked close to sixty miles to enlist.
> He had weak lungs but he passed the medical and got to go to the front lines.
> (McLean, 2005, pp. 28–29)

I reflected, too, on my mother, my grandfather's daughter, who had herself been a geriatric head nurse, soldiering on for long hours at the hospital psychiatric wards and caring for patients for more than 30 years. Many of the people she cared for ended their lives at the hospital. I interviewed my mother, "Irene," who told me one of her nursing assignments had been to dispense medications like tranquilizers and phenobarbital to 450 older patients, twice daily, on five wards.

In the "geriatric nurse" scene, I act out the story of my mother carrying out her duties at the hospital in 1964. Later, I perform her role in the present, a retired nurse, now 76 years old, at home in her own bed and unable to sleep as she remembers her experiences with dying patients. She wonders how she will be treated at the end of her own life. During this scene, an audio recording of my mother's voice is played over the speakers for the audience. The lines she delivered from the script were drawn from my interviews with my mother as she expressed her concerns about choices and decision making when one is dying in hospital.

IRENE:
In the journey of life much planning goes into milestone events
such as marriages, anniversaries and even funerals …
dying is the one event impossible to preplan
although every living thing dies.
Place yourself in the position of your afflicted client and consider,
what freedom will I have to assert my rights for a dignified end?
If rational and aware of my own situation
will my wishes regarding my management be heard and communicated?
If I can no longer act for myself
who will determine those measures meant to prolong my life
and ease the dying process? (McLean, 2005, pp. 26–27)

My mother's questions reflect the deepest of human fears, and the scene presents an embodied, empathic role reversal of the caregiver–patient position. If we are dying in hospital, lying in that bed, who will determine how we die or whether we will suffer?

One day, while visiting the hospital to do some more research, I stopped at the cafeteria for my usual cup of coffee. I had nearly completed the script but was looking for some way to conclude, to end on a hopeful note that might point toward change. That was when I bought that last coffee from the volunteer behind the counter. His name was Jacob. Jacob had served my coffee many times when I'd visited the hospital cafeteria, usually with a little advice. He was 87 years old and a survivor of Auschwitz. I asked him if he had a spoon.

"Never want for another's spoon," he had said, "but hold on to your own spoon very carefully."

I will never forget Jacob's words.

The spoon, precious as life, held tight by survivors.

Illuminated metaphorically, the spoon in this performance represented autonomy, personhood, hope and life itself. This was, for me, an epiphany. Even when facing death and terrible adversity, there is still hope if we hold tight to what we believe in. I incorporated the story of that meeting with Jacob and his wise words about the spoon into one of the final scenes of the ethnodrama.

Results: First Production

In the lecture hall at the Rene Cassin Institute of Social Gerontology, 30 social workers, nurses, clinicians and researchers gathered to see *Remember me for birds.* I discovered that this performance raised awareness about issues of older people's mental health and autonomy and, further, that audience members found the performance had a lasting impact and increased their learning.

All but five audience members indicated they experienced some change in terms of understanding client autonomy as a direct result of this performance. The five who commented that they did not experience change observed that the overall performance accurately reflected their own experiences and what they knew, and felt it validated their clients' experience. All but three people who attended responded more favourably to a performance than to a lecture; most attendees found the performance vividly highlighted the fact that everyone is an individual, and it moved them emotionally more than a lecture would. This result substantiates the strategy to choose performance as a useful form of communication with health care workers to help raise awareness about issues that affect autonomy for older people.

The coordinator of the mental-health program remarked,

> The quality of autonomy was given "life." Despite over 20 years working in the field of gerontology, this performance embraced the very basics of life that those younger take for granted. This was a "window to their souls." Excellent! Should be presented for incoming social workers and could be used for orientation. A lasting impact!

A social worker observed,

> Highlights the essence of a human being which remains throughout the years. These people are calling out for help and understanding. A performance zeros in

> on the deepest emotions and allows the viewer to gain a deep understanding of the person's pain, joy. Through drama, barriers to understanding are broken down.

An elder-abuse researcher who attended expressed a sense of transformation and personal learning:

> There is a paternalism with regard to the elderly. This often results in their autonomy being assumed to be less than it is or taken away against their will. I learned I am inappropriately detached from people. I came. I attended because I was curious and I am glad I came. I learned about others but it [the performance] taught me about myself.

The educative element was important to many audience members. One social worker described her experience as follows: "The vivid expression (performance) helps one to empathize and to relate more humanely to the person as opposed to treating the issue as another body of knowledge." Another audience member said, "The insight it brings, the emotions felt during the ethnodrama will affect insights and orientations in our practices."

Since the original research performance, and after the ethnodrama had evolved into an hour-long, full production, I have continued to perform *Remember me for birds* for universities and health organizations in Canada and the United States. A DVD of *Remember me for birds* was made and has been screened for audiences at numerous keynotes and presentations related to the creative arts in interdisciplinary research and practice.

It may not always be possible, nor practical, for medical educators, students and other allied health professionals to research, write and launch a full ethnodrama. Still, using dramatic approaches or creative arts methods with groups as a means to offer places for story and self-expression can be helpful.

For example, in my ongoing workshops for professional health care providers, Living Stories of Hope and Change, I use the creative arts in action well beyond simple physician–patient role-plays and patient simulations. Health professionals across hierarchies and disciplines are introduced to story through group work, using a developmental process that draws from creative-arts methods such as collage making, role-play, embodiment and drama. This introduction brings participants to a place of readiness to express and write their own narratives and personal monologues. Along with sharing stories of their work and personal lives, participants take part in a process of deep self-discovery, where listening is fostered as a vital skill for understanding the richness of the human story and experiences are validated in a caring, supportive environment. The sessions culminate in a group performance for witnesses. Over time we have welcomed to our circles emergency-room physicians, nurses who work in palliative care, mental-health counsellors, social workers, chaplains and dietitians, among others.

Conclusion

An ethnodrama performance can raise awareness, educating well beyond the podium, conveying lived experience in action with visual,

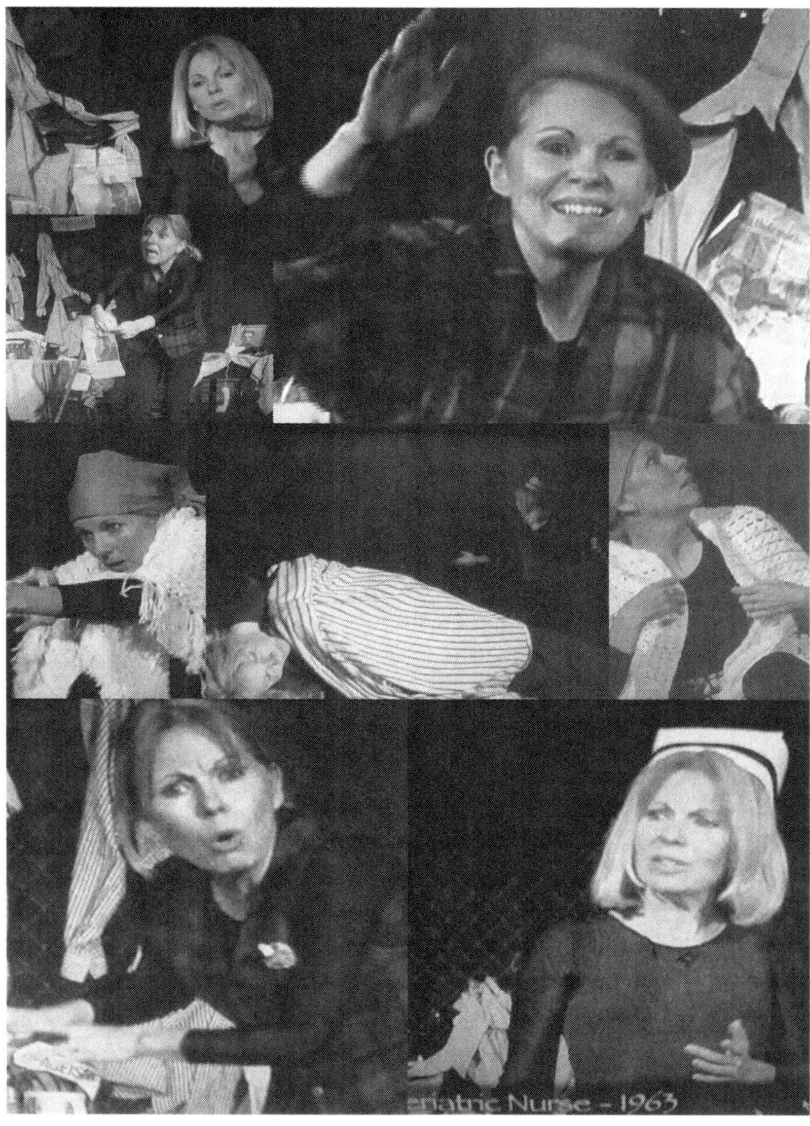

Figure 2.3 A photo collage of scenes from *Remember me for birds*

emotional, physical and spiritual elements. It is a field process whereby we are told and we tell stories, engaging in one of the most meaningful and universal of human connections.

I had set out in my research to create a performance based on true stories and lived experience that would raise awareness about autonomy and mental health by re-illuminating stories people working in health care experience every day in their work in aging and health. If I could not, in an immediate sense, bring people to action, I hoped through this performance to transform the way people think about older people. This was, I believed, where change would begin: in care that would contribute to quality of life from day to day for people at home, in residential care or in long-term-care facilities. It might also help in reforming health care policy that can have a direct bearing on well-being, autonomy and consequently the mental health of all those whom the system should be adequately designed to serve. After all, some 40 million people in the United States are currently age 65 or older, and this number is expected to climb to 89 million by 2050.

Active and performative research methods have much to offer education and health, with new ways for medical educators, students and others in the allied health professions to learn about aging and humane medicine. Through performance and what the arts can offer, caregivers have the opportunity to develop greater awareness, empathy and understanding, which could improve quality of life for us all. It is, I believe, an offering of hope that we should treasure and hold on to very carefully.

NOTES

I would like to acknowledge Yehudit Silverman, Creative Arts Therapies, Concordia University, for her encouragement and support during the formative stages of this performance.

1 Saldaña shares a selected literature review of 38 ethnodramatic play scripts about health and illness on topics such as women's breast cancer, prostate cancer and effects on men and spouses, surviving ovarian cancer, a gay man's struggle with cancer, physician and cancer patient communication, living without health insurance, and nursing-home care, among others. See Saldaña, 2010.

REFERENCES

Charon, R. (2008). *Narrative medicine: Honoring the stories of illness.* New York: Oxford University Press.

Denzin, N.K. (2003). *Performance ethnography, critical pedagogy and the politics of culture.* Thousand Oaks, CA: Sage Publications.

Gibran, K. (1966). *The wisdom of Gibran.* New York: Philosophical Library.

Gold, M. (2000). *Therapy through drama: The fictional family.* Springfield, IL: Charles C. Thomas.

McLean, C.L. (2005). *Remember me for birds: An ethnodrama about aging, mental health and autonomy (script book).* Cochrane, AB: Ravenquest Inc.

Saldaña, J. (2005). *Ethnodrama: An anthology of reality theatre.* Walnut Creek, CA: AltaMira Press.

Saldaña, J. (2010). Ethnodramas about health and illness: Staging human vulnerability, fragility and resiliency. In C.L. McLean & R. Kelly (Eds.), *Creative arts in interdisciplinary practice: Inquiries for hope and change* (pp. 167–184). Calgary, AB: Detselig Enterprises.

Saldaña, J. (2011). *Ethnotheatre: Research from page to stage.* Walnut Creek, CA: Left Coast Press.

Lifelines

The Art of Medicine Challenges the Humanity Within Us

Craig Chen, MD

No matter how much physicians try to resist the notion, a lot of medicine has an algorithmic, cookbook or heuristic nature. I dislike this idea. We wish to think the art of medicine magical, as if our years of training, nights poring over books, experiences with thousands of patients and Socratic teaching method impart on us some wisdom that allows us to lay hands on a patient and diagnose. But the truth is that rapidly improving technologies, faster computational algorithms, advances in machine learning and the complexity of human wellness and disease mean that computers have begun to challenge even the most experienced and well-respected physicians. Physicians dislike patients who come to appointments carrying printouts from Google searches of their symptoms, yet we cannot deny that our clinical expertise can often be matched by technology.

That being said, I still believe the art of medicine is an art that challenges the humanity within us. Emotions, stories, artwork, reflection, discussion and debate challenge us to hone our skills of taking care of the *person.* A computer may make the diagnosis, but a physician broaches the delivery of that diagnosis and cultivates the relationship of trust necessary for compassionate care. We don't respect that skill set enough. It is not easy to go to work every day and care for people who hurt themselves, are going to die, cry on your shoulder, feel terrified or distrust the health care system. With respect to medicine, the arts and humanities help us understand how humans experience illness and disease, and place that experience in a context of diagnosis, treatment and care.

3

The Visual Arts in Health Education at the Melbourne Dental School

Mina Borromeo, Heather Gaunt and Neville Chiavaroli

The Visual Arts in Health Education (VAHE) program, based at the Ian Potter Museum of Art (IPMoA) at the University of Melbourne, was initiated in 2012. Like many programs successfully conducted in universities in the United States and elsewhere, this program builds on the shared expertise of staff in both the visual arts and health education. The IPMoA seminars are facilitated by a combination of clinicians, art academics and/or educationalists and involve two-hour sessions at the museum. During these seminars, students are guided to observe and interpret artworks on display in exhibitions to practice their skills of visual observation, develop their empathic understanding and think about and learn from art in the context of their profession. The VAHE program was developed initially for senior medical students at the University of Melbourne in their palliative care training at a specialist cancer hospital, the Peter MacCallum Cancer Centre. In this article we report on its use as part of the teaching of special-needs dentistry (SND) to graduate students in the university's Doctor of Clinical Dentistry and Doctor of Dental Surgery courses.

Value of Arts-Based Training in Health Professionals' Education

Evidence for the value of arts-based training in health professionals' education is accumulating. There is now high-quality evidence

(Perry, Maffulli, Willson & Morrissey, 2011) for improvement in students' general observation skills as a result of viewing and discussing artworks, with several studies indicating a transfer to the clinical context (Dolev, Friedlaender & Braverman, 2001; Naghshineh et al., 2008; Braverman, 2011). In some cases, the evidence for change is anecdotal (Perry, Maffulli, Willson & Morrissey, 2011), but some findings suggest that engaging systematically with art in facilitated and collaborative contexts may improve students' capacity to focus on and infer emotions (Bardes, Gillers & Herman, 2001), raise awareness and sensitivity to patients in medical contexts (Reilly, Ring & Duke, 2005), and increase emotional awareness in others and self (Shapiro, Rucker & Beck, 2006). The importance of empathy in clinical practice has been shown by numerous studies (as reviewed by Stepien & Baernstein, 2006).

Although arts-based interventions have been shown to improve core clinical skills in medical curricula, their use in facilitating clinical observation and improving empathy as part of dental curricula is lacking (Bardes, Gillers & Herman, 2001; Naghshineh et al., 2008). The role of visual-art interventions blended with traditional didactic teaching using photographs and clinical scenarios has been reported to be beneficial as part of medical training (Shapiro et al., 2006).

In a broad sense, the arts are increasingly recognized as an effective means of facilitating the development of empathy in health professionals and have given rise to a thriving discipline known for many years as the medical humanities, now referred to increasingly as the health humanities. The idea of facilitating the development of observational skills and empathy through such indirect approaches as the observation and interpretation of art has gained further support from other developments in health professional pedagogy. The methods currently in use for facilitating visual thinking share key elements and principles with problem-based learning, a teaching approach widely adopted over the past three decades in health professional curricula and based on active, collaborative, contextual and self-directed learning (Savery, 2006). As discussed below, these elements resonate with visual thinking approaches currently employed in art museums and arts faculties to foster student learning in the areas outlined above.

Teaching Special-Needs Dentistry at the University of Melbourne

The original VAHE seminar, given in the context of palliative care, aimed to introduce students to skills in visual analysis specifically to enhance their clinical diagnostic skills. This pilot program was introduced in the second half of 2012 into the Melbourne Dental School. The convener of special-needs dentistry recognized that a similar approach could be used to enhance the teaching of this sub-specialty to dental students. The program was piloted with a small group of post-graduate trainee specialists, with some modifications to the approach used with medical students. A key focus for the program was to address issues related to empathy in the context of individuals with special needs, an aspect that was not explicitly taught in other components of the dental curriculum at either preclinical or clinical stages. Hence the program for the SND students focused heavily on discussing subjective aspects of students' observations of works of art on display in the museum, followed by explicit links to the field of SND with an emphasis on articulating the narratives suggested by the artworks and the development of empathic understanding (Yarascavitch, Regehr, Hodges & Haas, 2009).

Special-needs dentistry is defined as that part of dentistry associated with the management of the oral health of individuals who are medically compromised, have intellectual or physical disabilities or have psychiatric problems (Royal Australasian College of Dental Surgeons [RACDS], 2009). It has also been recognized by the World Health Organization in the context of the International Classification of Functioning involving those with a disability or activity restriction that directly or indirectly affects their oral health, within the personal and environmental context of the individual (World Health Organization, 2001; Faulks & Hennequin, 2006). In Australia, SND has been recognized as a specialty since 2002 and is taught in most dental schools at an undergraduate and graduate level, and in three universities at the post-graduate level. This discipline, like others, competes for space in a tight curriculum at the undergraduate level.

It can be easy to forget that the tooth is part of the mouth and the mouth is part of the face, which is connected to the rest of the body. All too often students are so heavily focused on what they need to know to pass the next examination that they lose sight of the fact that they are managing the oral-health needs of an individual and, in the case of special-needs dentistry, of an individual with complex needs. As important as the foundational knowledge is, it may well lead to forgetting the essence of the profession, a health discipline involved in improving people's quality of life.

The focus of teaching in dentistry in Australia is changing, with a greater emphasis being placed on interdisciplinary and interprofessional approaches to care and a move toward consideration of the whole patient rather than discrete aspects of oral health, such as the teeth or the periodontal structures. People with complex medical, behavioural, psychological and/or psychiatric issues may not be recognized as having special needs. The category of patients frequently omitted is the elderly. Given that we are living in an aging population, this omission is concerning. Moreover, there are disparities between those with special needs and the ability of the dental workforce to meet their demands (Lawton 2002; Ettinger, Chalmers & Frenkel, 2004; Albino, Inglehart & Tedesco, 2012). In Australia alone, there are over 1.2 million individuals with profound or severe core-activity limitations, and thus the number of those with special needs ranging from minor to severe is much greater; yet there are only 13 registered specialists in SND (Australian Bureau of Statistics [ABS], 2003). This gap further highlights the need for interventions aimed at improving empathy and communication skills at the undergraduate or graduate level to equip all dental graduates with the skills to address these disparities within the profession (Lawton 2002; Albino, Inglehart & Tedesco, 2012)—particularly as evidence suggests that empathy may decline during health professional training and clinical practice (Hojat, Gonnella, Nasca, Mangione, Vergare & Magee, 2002; Sherman and Cramer 2005; Yarascavitch et al., 2009).

The VAHE program was conceived as one way of redressing this situation. One of the key aims was to improve students' ability to notice relevant information. For example, when asked what they see when they look at someone in a wheelchair, students commonly respond, the wheelchair. It often takes considerable discussion to look past the physical barrier of the wheelchair. Some dental students will see the mouth or the state of the teeth, but rarely will they report on the individual in the wheelchair, his/her clothing, objects hanging from the wheelchair that may relate to the personality of the individual or items such as a walking stick that may signify some degree of mobility beyond the wheelchair.

Similarly, students' learning about patient empathy begins with an understanding of the individual before them. Empathy has been defined conventionally with two components: affective (emotional) and cognitive (Duan & Hill, 1996). The former involves sharing or taking on another's emotional state, while the latter refers to the more intellectual process of seeing another's perspective, or at least understanding another's thoughts and feelings. While both aspects might conceivably benefit from systematic viewing and interpretation of (representational) artworks, health professional educators generally agree that cognitive empathy is the more appropriate form in clinical situations (Halpern, 2001) and is normally the target of educational interventions. Teaching students to analyze artworks objectively and subjectively, away from their usual environment and in a setting not associated with the high expectations and intellectual and emotional challenges of the clinical world, can provide a useful first step.

The VAHE Program for Students of Special-Needs Dentistry

The VAHE program was first delivered to the full second-year cohort of 84 doctors of dental surgery students as a component of the SND curriculum from July to November 2012, over several single sessions. Each session lasted two hours and consisted of students working in pairs, with each pair assigned a separate artwork. The program aimed to foster the development of systematic and coherent ways of seeing, and effective communication of what had been seen. The particular method used is closely based on the Harvard model pioneered by Irwin Braverman (2011) and more broadly informed by the work of Housen (2001). VAHE seminars were structured around the key elements of objective observation, subjective interpretation, reflection and discussion within the group, and finally explicit and facilitated application to clinical situations. This process is represented in Figure 3.1.

Selection of Artworks

All artworks for the program were selected from paintings in the University of Melbourne art collections currently on display in an exhibition entitled *The anatomy lesson*, which was created to celebrate the 40th anniversary of the university's art museum. The artworks chosen for analysis featured specific elements with which empathic understanding could be enhanced in the context of special-needs dentistry. Several features determined our choice of artworks for the SND seminar. The first was that the human or anthropomorphically suggestive element needed to be a central feature of the artwork, since a key objective was students' development of empathy for and understanding of patients with special needs. Second, sufficient detail was needed to support a rich objective analysis to promote the students' visual observation skills. Third, the artwork should contain suggestive or ambiguous elements to allow students scope to imagine different scenarios to explain the narrative of the artwork. An overtly realistic image with a self-evident narrative may have left students unused to visual interpretation with little opportunity for interpretation, even though in practice it has been our experience that most artworks do in fact lend themselves to some

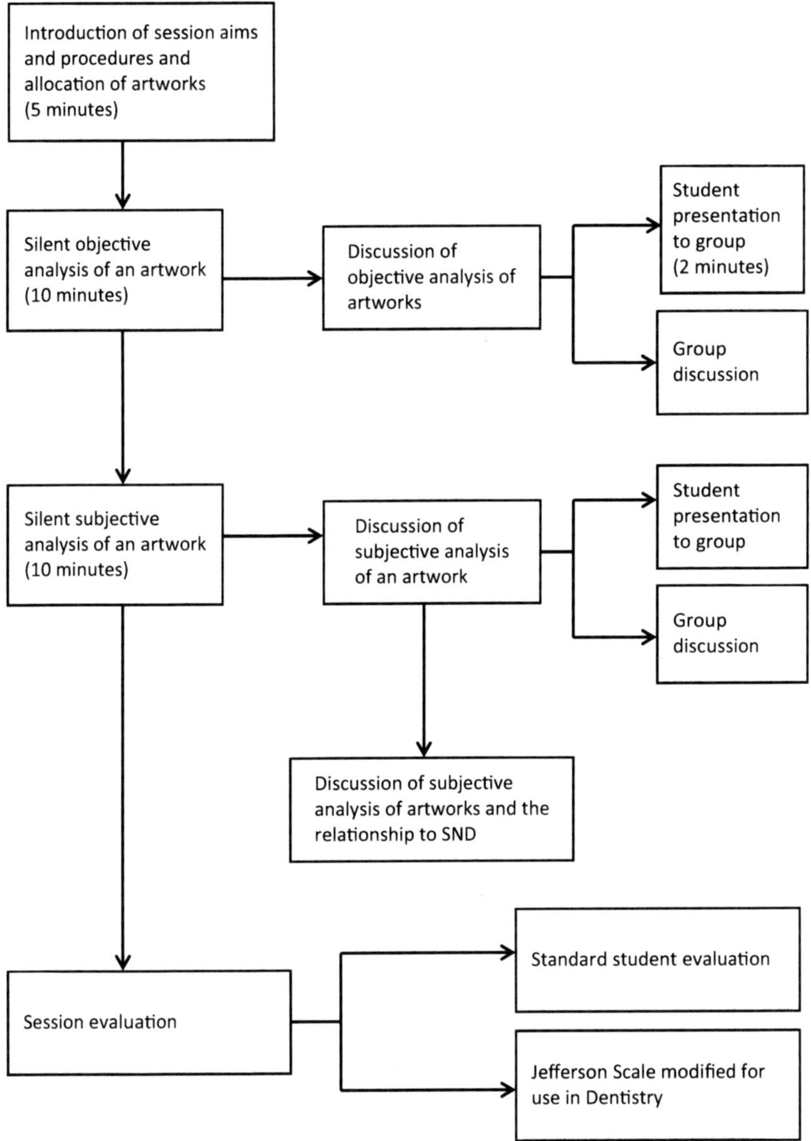

Figure 3.1 Flow diagram of VAHE session outline for second-year dental students

form of narrative interpretation. Within these parameters, artworks from a variety of subject matter, media and periods were selected to stimulate further debate and comparisons between works.

All information concerning the artist and title of the artworks was withheld from the students until the end of the session, to encourage close visual analysis of the work itself rather than an authoritative reference. Program staff circulated among the students, encouraging and facilitating their observations and interpretations. This encouragement commonly consisted of reassurance that there was no right or wrong answer and that it was their ability to observe closely and imagine the underlying story that was the focus of session.

Objective Analysis

The aim in this first phase was to encourage students to look closely at the artwork and practice the ability to notice as much detail as possible. Students were primed to observe closely and relate accurately with prompts such as "describe what you see to someone who cannot see the painting." Students were discouraged from attempting to interpret meaning during this phase. The task was primarily to observe and report back to the group with a detailed description of the assigned artwork.

An example of an artwork particularly appropriate to this type of objective analysis was the visually complex painting *The queen* (1988) by John Brack. Students were encouraged to work progressively from macro to micro analysis, looking for patterns and connections between visual elements, such as repeated shapes (e.g., ovals, rectangles), the layering of picture planes and the way the eye was drawn to different areas of the painting by vertical stripes in the background. Facilitators stressed that rich visual observation involves looking not once but many times and puzzling over the data that had been gathered. The aim was to begin to instill in students the need to look many times before closing their minds to what they saw. Students were also encouraged to be alert to conflicting or ambiguous visual information. In *The queen*, for example, discussion centred on the visual uncertainty generated by the table leg that leads the eye downwards but is cut off at the edge of the wallpaper. Students also considered the figure as a whole and the visual relationships of the postcards and their mirrored images. Visual analyses typically included details such as the fractured pieces of the female figure, her costume and jewelry, and the number, shape, size, orientation and pertinent placement of the scissors on the table.

Subjective Analysis

The objective observation phase of each session was followed by a subjective analysis of the same artwork. Students were encouraged to interpret the visual data they had gathered in the objective analysis and establish what they believed was the story within the artwork, referring back to what they had seen. Students were also encouraged to explore how the artwork made them feel and to identify what aspect of the artwork elicited these emotional responses, as a way of helping them understand the narrative within the artwork. Typically these responses related to the way the human figures were depicted or to specific visual elements such as size, colour and texture.

For example, students' subjective interpretations of *The queen* focused on the image of the woman at the centre. They concluded she was wealthy and possibly royal, given her dress and pose. Students interpreted the fracturing of her image as suggesting distorted self-perception (noting the function of the mirror) or psychological instability. The scissors were identified as the cause of this disruption, yet at the same time also interpreted anthropomorphically, considering the way they were grouped in a familial hierarchical structure with larger scissors (parents) at the centre and the smaller scissors (children) flanking and placed further back on the picture plane, and a single figure lying prone in the foreground. Students also considered the emotive effect of these non-human but humanized visual elements; for example, the fracturing of the woman's image prompted them to feel disjunction and a sense of unhappiness and unease.

Students' engagement in this interpretive phase of the program was striking. It was evident that for many it was where the most stimulating and potentially transformative educational experience was occurring. Central to the experience was a sense of freedom: there was no right or wrong answer and no final expert opinion to be learned. Rather, there was repeated opportunity to speculate and debate visual clues and narrative interpretation and to touch on relevance to real-world practice, irrespective of whether the artwork was depicting the imagined circumstances or not. The freedom to observe, interpret and engage in in-depth discussions allowed students to focus beyond simple dental aspects of clinical relevance onto the personal, qualitative world of the individuals—and potential future patients—represented in the artworks.

It was possible for students to engage in this visual-thinking process even with artworks far removed from their daily experience—for example, the 16th-century print *St Jerome* by Lucas van Leyden, which depicts a physical environment far removed from 21st-century life and replete with Christian iconography. Deliberately eschewing these historical and iconographic aspects, students were encouraged to describe only what they saw: the human figure, his age, pose, clothing, surrounding objects, the physical environment and so on. They also came to appreciate the need to revisit first impressions of an artwork (and by extension a patient) to ensure important elements were not overlooked, such as the hat hanging on the box, a detail often missed by students during the objective analysis phase. Where students missed such detail, they were encouraged to look again, to note—and report—the presence of the apparently insignificant.

Again, the subjective analysis provided the opportunity to explore the relative significance and meaning of the different elements in the picture. The group sought to understand, for example, whether or not the hat (once noted) played an important role in the figure characterization. Similarly, students debated the meaning of the skull (emphasized for the viewer by the figure's pointing finger), considering possibilities that the figure was dwelling on the idea of mourning, approaching death or perhaps immortality. The area of light behind the figure's head was commonly identified as a halo in Christian iconography, suggesting possible sainthood of the figure, and a strong Christian theme was further evidenced by the crucifix in the figure's grasp. As some students were not familiar with such Christian imagery, seminar facilitators provided information as necessary, such as the fact that the hat was in fact a cardinal's hat, indicating the status of the figure. However, such information could narrow the focus and prematurely close the interpretation, although it also led to discussions about encultured ways of seeing and the parallels in communication and diagnoses in health care situations, where health practitioners need to be aware of their own encultured responses and potential biases.

Application in the Context of Special-Needs Dentistry

For the dental students, the final step of engaging with the paintings involved drawing direct connections with the human elements in the artworks and projecting these into possible clinical scenarios. Here facilitators guided the conversation, drawing attention to key elements that might have parallels in their eventual clinical practice. For example, might the facial expression and bodily pose in the *St Jerome* portrait suggest depression, despair, hunger or even dementia in an elderly patient? If the patient suffered dementia, the clinician would need to consider what the patient could accomplish for himself, how much autonomy the patient would have and how much help he would require from caregivers. If the patient were an alcoholic, would he be able to maintain dental health, and would he be more likely to have many cavities or a high extraction rate? Could he afford dental treatment or the cost of a toothbrush and toothpaste? If he suffered from other illnesses, dentistry might be very low on his health priorities.

Students were encouraged to discuss how they would manage each of these various scenarios raised as a result of observation, discussion and engagement with this artwork.

Another compelling artwork from the perspective of the application phase was Henry Moore's *Untitled (family group).* After the objective analysis phase, most students were not only able but keen to posit alternative narratives about the figures depicted and their dynamics and relationships

The seated girl by Hugh Ramsay provided a different challenge. Students had the opportunity to focus their visual analyses on an artwork that was apparently simpler in content and portrayed the solitary figure of a young girl seen from behind. Here, objective analysis brought out very rich descriptions of skin and hair quality, pose and posture, body composition and dress. Subjective interpretations then considered possible personal narratives for the girl, with students considering why she might not be showing her face; many students offered emotional responses to the portrait. Students were encouraged to identify and describe which specific visual elements elicited particular emotional responses, and they commented about specifying the colours used by the artist in the background, the pose, the slope of the shoulders and the slightly messy hair. Some students noted that the figure seemed sad or dejected—an interesting response given that the figure's face was not observable. This response initially surprised many, but also appeared to reflect the students' engagement and growing confidence in interpreting the artworks. In then applying their responses to the SND context, students discussed such issues as the impact of an eating disorder on dental health and gaining the trust of patient with increased sensitivities—especially if invasive treatment was necessary.

It should be clear from the above examples that the SND sessions are less concerned with direct transfer to the context of clinical reasoning than other visual-thinking programs, including others conducted as part of the VAHE program at the IPMoA (such as the original program run with palliative care students). Where other programs might emphasize the transferability of the skills practiced during the objective and subjective phases to the clinical context (Bardes et al., 2001; Naghshineh et al., 2008; Braverman, 2011), the key objective for the SND students was to enhance understanding and empathy for what it might mean to be a special-needs patient. Accordingly, more time was spent on encouraging and facilitating students to tap into the emotional impact of the images and/or imagining possible underlying narratives behind the images of people.

Student Engagement and Responses

The degree of student engagement in the two-hour seminars was palpable and very exciting for the teachers, particularly as such an approach had not been previously used in the context of SND at our university. Over the course of the multiple iterations of the seminar, consistent engagement was clearly displayed by most students. Unprompted statements during the seminar included the casually enthusiastic (and somewhat surprised) "this is fun," which, while not reflecting a specific learning objective, indicated that a positive connection had been made between the student and the learning environment. This comment was all the more satisfying when expressed by students who had been initially circumspect, if not openly sceptical. Some students admittedly found the art aspect difficult to relate to the dental aspect, while others found this the most interesting and preferred part of the session. Students also generally appreciated the opportunity to engage in subjective and speculative discussion to identify hidden meaning, using essentially unfamiliar material. One student noted the most relevant and stimulating aspect to be the

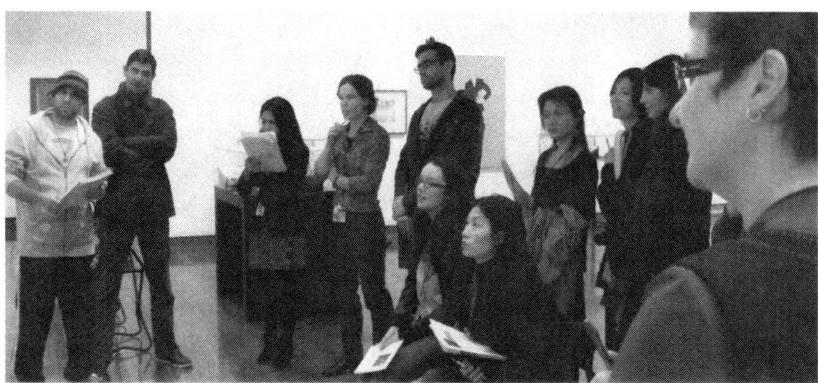

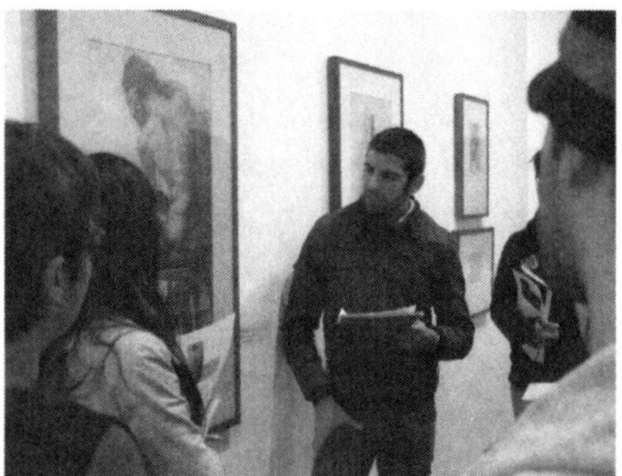

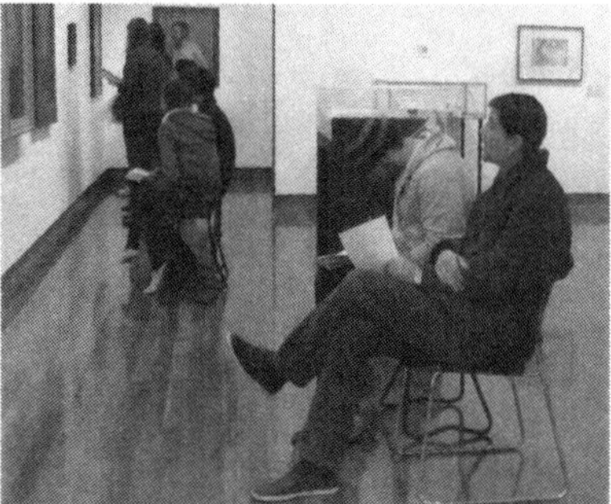

Figure 3.2 Special-needs dentistry students during a VAHE session

"discussion amongst instructors, different ideas, discussion from how people look differently at the same subject of work." Another student appreciated the "links between humanity and health." Others felt the relevance was not immediately apparent but still found the discussion of clinical concerns using art as a medium interesting.

Students embraced the emotive aspects of the seminar in particular, one noting as a highlight the "strong emotional content." Occasionally this aspect affected students directly; for example, one student became tearful while discussing a possible autism scenario. The student chose to share that she had a young family member similarly affected, and this disclosure prompted further empathy and compassion in her peers and a discussion of how emotions have a significant role in clinical work beyond "performing a single filling."

Student Evaluation of the Session

All the dental students found the sessions valuable and reported that they had learned new skills in visual observation (both objective and subjective) and that training in the visual arts enhanced their training in special needs. It had also improved their empathy for special-needs dental patients. They reported the sessions to be stimulating. One graduate student reported that "analysing the individuals and their expressions [as portrayed in the artworks] was a key tool for dentists in everything for the patients. Subjective analysis is critical for patient treatment especially in special-needs dentistry." Thus, we are able to demonstrate that the VAHE sessions engaged students and had an overall positive effect, at least in the short term, on their self-reported levels of empathy.

Reflections and Challenges

The facility and willingness with which students were able to enter the imaginary spaces of the artworks underpin for us the value of this method of teaching, for encouraging students to think outside their field of health education in ways that will enrich their abilities to work in that field.

In our view, the location of this program within the museum environment is also a critical feature of its potential success. To view the artworks on paper or projected on a screen may at times be a necessary compromise, but the opportunity to engage with the art at actual size and displayed as intended brings a vividness and immediacy that we find is otherwise lacking. As well, the effect of separation from the usual pedagogic environment of the lecture theatre, tutorial room or science laboratory should not be underestimated.

Clearly there are several challenges when designing and implementing this type of program. Inevitably, considerations involve the most appropriate artworks to select, the most appropriate format for the sessions, how best to link artworks to dental clinical scenarios and how best to fit the program into the already tight timetable or overcrowded curriculum, among others.

During the subjective and clinical application phases, it is important to allow students the space and safe environment to express their views, no matter how seemingly implausible or lateral they may appear initially. Facilitators or fellow students can and should query some interpretations to prompt the student to focus on identifiable aspects of the artwork or to better understand the basis of the interpretation. This needs to be done in a collaborative and supportive way. The different teaching environment should not mean that the normal protocols of collaborative (and active) learning expected and facilitated in other contexts, such as problem-based learning tutorials, are ignored in the museum.

The idea of using artworks for the teaching of SND was initially met with scepticism by many students and staff in the dental school. It was clear, however, that students enjoyed the experience and that it generated interest among staff, culminating in a trial session with dental staff. There are many challenges ahead as this program is developed across the dental school and the university at large. Clearly there needs to be further and more systematic assessment of the program, not only so that evidence regarding its potential long-term benefits can be obtained but also to allow growth of the program beyond a single session to a long-term medical humanities program that we hope will ultimately benefit overall patient care.

A further challenge to the program is how most effectively to transfer and consolidate the learning achieved in the single museum seminar. Currently we can only offer single seminars to various student groups because of the inevitable demands on the dental curriculum. In contrast, similar programs in the United States typically consist of a series of up to eight museum seminars, reinforcing visual-observation skills through repetition and practice (Bardes et al., 2001; Naghshineh et al., 2008). Student feedback on the seminars to date indicates many of our students desire repeat sessions and a greater availability of the arts observational program.

Our early experience with the VAHE approach to teaching SND students therefore suggests that not only is the general approach sound, but the method used is effective and flexible. The artwork provides a rich prompt for thought and discussion, both in isolation and in the context of SND, while remaining free of its historical, cultural or technical properties. The objective analysis creates the opportunity for clear insight, the subjective analysis allows communication with the human side (in other words, empathy) and the final phase represents the applied or symbolic interpretation in the SND context—that is, a way of making the lessons learned explicit and therefore transferable. In so doing, students are guided through the rediscovery and re-appreciation of the place and value of basic human responses in health education in general, and in the specific context of special-needs dentistry.

REFERENCES

Albino, J.E., Inglehart, M.R., & Tedesco, L.A. (2012, Jan). Dental education and changing oral health care needs: disparities and demands. *Journal of Dental Education, 76*(1), 75–88. Medline:22262552

Australian Bureau of Statistics [ABS] (2003). *Disability, Ageing and Carers, Australia: Summary of Findings*. Retrieved from http://www.ausstats.abs.gov.au/ausstats/

Bardes, C.L., Gillers, D., & Herman, A.E. (2001, Dec). Learning to look: developing clinical observational skills at an art museum. *Medical Education, 35*(12), 1157–1161. http://dx.doi.org/10.1046/j.1365-2923.2001.01088.x Medline:11895244

Braverman, I.M. (2011, May-Jun). To see or not to see: how visual training can improve observational skills. *Clinics in Dermatology, 29*(3), 343–346. http://dx.doi.org/10.1016/j.clindermatol.2010.08.001 Medline:21496744

Dolev, J.C., Friedlaender, L.K., & Braverman, I.M. (2001, Sep 5). Use of fine art to enhance visual diagnostic skills. *Journal of the American Medical Association, 286*(9), 1020–1021. http://dx.doi.org/10.1001/jama.286.9.1020 Medline:11559280

Duan, C., & Hill, C.E. (1996). The current state of empathy research. *Journal of Counseling Psychology, 43*(3), 261–274. http://dx.doi.org/10.1037/0022-0167.43.3.261

Ettinger, R.L., Chalmers, J., & Frenkel, H. (2004, Aug). Dentistry for persons with special needs: how should it be recognized? *Journal of Dental Education, 68*(8), 803–806. Medline:15286100

Faulks, D., & Hennequin, M. (2006). Defining the population requiring special care dentistry using the International Classification of Functioning, Disability and Health—a personal view. *Journal of Disability and Oral Health*, 7(3), 143–152

Halpern, J. (2001). *From detached concern to empathy: Humanizing medical practice*. New York: Oxford University Press.

Hojat, M., Gonnella, J.S., Nasca, T.J., Mangione, S., Vergare, M., & Magee, M. (2002, Sep). Physician empathy: definition, components, measurement, and relationship to gender and specialty. *American Journal of Psychiatry, 159*(9), 1563–1569. http://dx.doi.org/10.1176/appi.ajp.159.9.1563 Medline:12202278

Housen, A. (2001, September). Eye of the beholder: Research, theory and practice. Paper presented at the conference: Aesthetic and Art Education: a transdisciplinary approach, Lisbon, Portugal.

Lawton, L. (2002, Dec). Providing dental care for special patients: tips for the general dentist. *Journal of the American Dental Association, 133*(12), 1666–1670. Medline:12512668

Naghshineh, S., Hafler, J.P., Miller, A.R., et al. (2008, Jul). Formal art observation training improves medical students' visual diagnostic skills. *Journal of General Internal Medicine, 23*(7), 991–997. http://dx.doi.org/10.1007/s11606-008-0667-0 Medline:18612730

Perry, M., Maffulli, N., Willson, S., & Morrissey, D. (2011, Feb). The effectiveness of arts-based interventions in medical education: a literature review. *Medical Education, 45*(2), 141–148. http://dx.doi.org/10.1111/j.1365-2923.2010.03848.x Medline:21208260

Reilly, J.M., Ring, J., & Duke, L. (2005, Apr). Visual thinking strategies: a new role for art in medical education. *Family Medicine, 37*(4), 250–252. Medline:15812693

Royal Australasian College of Dental Surgeons [RACDS] (2009). Definition of Special Needs Dentistry. Retrieved from: http://www.racds.org/examinations/special needs dentistry.

Savery, J.R. (2006). Overview of problem-based learning: Definitions and distinctions. *Interdisciplinary Journal of Problem-based Learning, 1*(1), 9–20. http://dx.doi.org/10.7771/1541-5015.1002

Shapiro, J., Rucker, L., & Beck, J. (2006, Mar). Training the clinical eye and mind: using the arts to develop medical students' observational and pattern recognition skills. *Medical Education, 40*(3), 263–268. http://dx.doi.org/10.1111/j.1365-2929.2006.02389.x Medline:16483329

Sherman, J.J., & Cramer, A. (2005, Mar). Measurement of changes in empathy during dental school. *Journal of Dental Education, 69*(3), 338–345. Medline:15749944

Stepien, K.A., & Baernstein, A. (2006, May). Educating for empathy. A review. *Journal of General Internal Medicine, 21*(5), 524–530. http://dx.doi.org/10.1111/j.1525-1497.2006.00443.x Medline:16704404

World Health Organization (WHO). (2001). *ICF: International Classification of Functioning, Disability and Health.* Geneva, Switzerland: World Health Organization.

Yarascavitch, C., Regehr, G., Hodges, B., & Haas, D.A. (2009, Apr). Changes in dental student empathy during training. *Journal of Dental Education, 73*(4), 509–517. Medline:19339438

SECTION 2

THE ARTS AND PRACTITIONER SELF-CARE

4

Advocating for Drama in Patient Communication

Alim Nagji, MD

As I peered past the thick black curtain, I could barely make out the audience amid the sea of harsh lights. From my hiding place in the wings of the vast auditorium, the stage seemed to stretch out toward infinity, the edges bleeding away in darkness. Only the shuffling of the patrons in their seats hinted at the boundary between my world and theirs. This is the theatre, where a storyteller captivates his audience with his story.

Waiting outside the room, demarcated only by a yellow-flowered sheet, I could hear the rustle within the room. The patient was shifting on the uncomfortable stretcher. As I entered, I squinted against the surgical light left on by the resident before me, greeted my patient and sat down. Her face was contorted in pain. Her arm grasped her left lower back as if by sheer force she could squelch away the source of her agony. Her eyes were sad and withdrawn; they flicked away quickly whenever I caught a glance head on. I waited for her story to begin.

There are numerous parallels between the theatre and medicine. At first they may seem worlds apart: one a farce, a parody of real life, where emotions are conjured and conflict staged, and the other filled with harsh realities, matters of life, death, disease and despair. In reality the two are intensely similar. The first requirement of theatre is that acting be real: the emotional commitment an actor makes is drawn from personal experiences, albeit under different circumstances. As an actor preparing for roles that were foreign to me, I often had to delve into the characters' back stories (Noice & Noice, 2002), drawing parallels between their experiences and my own to understand the decisions they made.

Teaching health professionals to understand their patients' stories must begin early in students' professional training, before their indoctrination into the cult of clinical practice leads to an erosion of empathy (Hojat et al., 2009). If we reach these students before clinical exposures, we can work with a clean slate and a willing audience. Over the past four years, an elective course of theatre-based exercises focused on communication skills has offered medical students an opportunity to reflect on their experiences as patients and providers. An ongoing collaborative arts—medicine program under Dr. Pamela Brett-MacLean, this elective was initially facilitated by Michael Kennard and has since developed and evolved under the expert direction of Michele Fleiger, both nationally recognized for their contributions to theatre. Offering a space for honest exploration, students are encouraged to channel their insights into future clinical encounters. One student commented:

> ... fear is what drives our inhibitions, and, to get over that, we need to just face it and go with our impulses and experience emotions that we might otherwise be embarrassed to display in front of others. That was a very useful thing that came out of it and I can definitely see how that can transpire over into the patient doctor relationship, where you can see how they might be fearing something and you can understand their point of view. I think that this theatrical exercise that we embarked upon definitely helped me to be able to see that. (Nagji & Brett-MacLean, 2013)

Honest communication must extend beyond patient encounters. In building relationships with their peers, health care professionals can find support networks to help withstand the host of stressors and responsibilities that can easily overwhelm them. Numerous studies have documented not only the high degree of stress but, more importantly, the poor coping mechanisms that may lead to higher rates of depression, alcoholism and, eventually, burnout (Dyrbye, Thomas & Shanafelt, 2006). Curricula rich in theatre-based exercises can be used to take down barriers and build lasting relationships among students, interdisciplinary groups and faculty; these relationships in turn can serve as protective mechanisms (Nagji, Brett-MacLean & Breault, in press; Dunn, Iglewicz & Moutier, 2008). As another student explains:

> I enjoyed it [the course] because although I've had a lot interpersonal activities pre-medically, [etc.], I feel like I was almost premature socially, because I had been

> involved in trying to get that GPA and that MCAT score, and, you know, the perfect application for medical school, that a lot of my own personal development had been delayed. I think I needed to do a lot of thinking about that and also think about how I valued relationships with other people. (Nagji, Brett-MacLean & Breault, 2013)

A variety of exercises are available from the dramatic arts to complement health care curricula. Drama games, for instance, can be used to break down rigid boundaries and equalize hierarchies, creating a fun, relaxing and welcoming atmosphere. Targeted exercises can be chosen to heighten awareness, such as *Making Contact*, where students glean the powers of observation and gain insight into their own non-verbal communication by making eye contact with each of their peers. Scene studies, based on students' own experiences, allow students to give voice to their emotional burdens and dissect new challenges they are facing. In larger classrooms, forum theatre can motivate students to reflect on creative solutions to common challenges, while workshopping their efficacy. Performances, which take students through the process of becoming characters and understanding scripts, can be used to explore ethical dilemmas and social norms (McCullough, 2012). The benefits of these and other humanities-based interventions have been described in the literature (Dow, Leong, Anderson & Wenzel, 2007; Kohn, 2011; Gordon, 2003; Reilly, Trial, Piver & Schaff, 2012).

The value in such exercises stems from breaking down the highly structured approach to learning that is typical of medical schools, reinvigorating students with a sense of "play" and reminding them of their own creativity and ability to accept ambiguity and uncertainty (Bleakley, 2012). These values can be brought about only in an experiential manner, as classroom- and lecture-based modules fail to prod students into active discovery.

> ... the sillier side of some of the ... games we played broke a lot of people out of their ... rigid like "I am a professional," ... like straight-cut edge ... It's OK to be silly ... by the end of it people were engaging each other, people were initiating that same kind of fun atmosphere ... I'm not saying get rid of your professionalism ... you maintain your professionalism but you still have a personality, you still have fun, you still make jokes, there's a time and place for everything. And so you still keep, like ... the respect that you have for each other as a person. ... (Nagji, Brett-MacLean & Breault, 2013)

Many educators may note the rise of simulation in medical education, from the Objective Structured Clinical Exams (OSCEs) in evaluation to standardized patient interviews in training. While simulation remains a cornerstone for certain areas of medicine, especially areas such as critical care and procedural skills, in the field of communication, authentic sharing is necessary lest students become adept at forged encounters by memorizing "empathetic" statements and displaying feigned compassion.

The key difference between usual approaches to role-playing in their educational programs and theatre-based exercises is that students remain keenly aware of the contrived nature of simulated interviews. Students will lament the shortcomings of their standardized patients, that they were too difficult or protective in divulging information. Theatre-based exercises focused on physician-patient communication involve students in taking on the role of both patients and physicians and reflecting on the interaction, which can enhance their ability to empathize. From our own research, quantitative changes in empathy can be seen after the completion of a theatre-based curriculum, demonstrating that empathy can be taught (Nagji & Brett-MacLean, 2011). Furthermore, this role reversal seeks to reinforce the central truth in medical care: all providers will eventually also be patients. This understanding further necessitates the formation and preservation of patient-centred modules.

In an age in which chronic diseases require a high degree of adherence to treatment, the therapeutic alliance between patients and their doctors is central to maintaining health. Merging theatre-based initiatives with core curriculum can have a meaningful impact on medical students' ability to maintain humanity, professionalism and compassion in their interviews, while also enhancing their resilience to stress and improving their well-being through the development of peer relationships. Moreover, these exercises can be used to build insight and reflective capacities, strengthening students' ability to recognize their own and their patients' emotions. Given that over half of the medical schools in the United States have already integrated arts-related activities (including performing arts) into their curricula (Rodenhauser, Strickland & Gambala, 2004), it is imperative that international curricula continue to develop and evaluate tailored programs for their students so as to train holistic, empathic health care professionals.

Though her story contained all the right details for me to make a diagnosis, it was the way in which she conveyed it that triggered me to think there were details being omitted. I paused frequently, letting silence descend heavily within the curtain, the department outside still in chaos. I offered comforting smiles, reassurances, and reaffirmed the confidentiality of our encounter. She made eye contact, and then I knew. When her narrative began, it was stuttering, full of caveats, and I worried that with each breath she may simply stop, but when she finished, she held my gaze. The curtain was drawn; the show was over.

REFERENCES

Bleakley, A. 2012. The health humanities: A democratizing force for medicine. In B. Sadler Takach, P. Brett-MacLean, & A. Rowe (Eds.), *InSight: Visualizing health humanities.* Edmonton, AB: Department of Art & Design, University of Alberta.

Dow, A.W., Leong, D., Anderson, A., Wenzel, R.P., & VCU Theater-Medicine Team. (2007, Aug). Using theater to teach clinical empathy: a pilot study. *Journal of General Internal Medicine, 22*(8), 1114–1118. http://dx.doi.org/10.1007/s11606-007-0224-2 Medline:17486385

Dunn, L.B., Iglewicz, A., & Moutier, C. (2008, Jan–Feb). A conceptual model of medical student well-being: promoting resilience and preventing burnout. *Academic Psychiatry, 32*(1), 44–53. http://dx.doi.org/10.1176/appi.ap.32.1.44 Medline:18270280

Dyrbye, L.N., Thomas, M.R., & Shanafelt, T.D. (2006, Apr). Systematic review of depression, anxiety, and other indicators of psychological distress among U.S. and Canadian medical students. *Academic Medicine, 81*(4), 354–373. http://dx.doi.org/10.1097/00001888-200604000-00009 Medline:16565188

Gordon, J. (2003, Apr). Fostering students' personal and professional development in medicine: a new framework for PPD. *Medical Education, 37*(4), 341–349. http://dx.doi.org/10.1046/j.1365-2923.2003.01470.x Medline:12654119

Hojat, M., Vergare, M.J., Maxwell, K., et al. (2009, Sep). The devil is in the third year: a longitudinal study of erosion of empathy in medical school. *Academic Medicine, 84*(9), 1182–1191. http://dx.doi.org/10.1097/ACM.0b013e3181b17e55 Medline:19707055

Kohn, M. (2011, Jun). Performing medicine: the role of theatre in medical education. *Medical Humanities, 37*(1), 3–4. http://dx.doi.org/10.1136/jmh.2011.007690 Medline:21593242

McCullough, M. (2012, Feb 11). Bringing drama into medical education. *Lancet, 379*(9815), 512–513. http://dx.doi.org/10.1016/S0140-6736(12)60221-9 Medline:22334885

Nagji, A., & Brett-MacLean, P. (2011). Acting in medicine: The role of theatre in teaching empathy. Poster at the Canadian Conference for Medical Education in Toronto, Ontario.

Nagji, A., & Brett-MacLean, P. Unpublished data (Focus Group VN620003, line 32–8, R4.).

Nagji, A., Brett-MacLean, P., & Breault, L. Exploring the benefits of an optional theatre module on medical student well-being. *Teaching and Learning in Medicine, 25*(3), 201–206. http://dx.doi.org/10.1080/10401334.2013.801774

Noice, T., & Noice, H. (2002). The expertise of professional actors: A review of recent research. *High Ability Studies, 13*(1), 7–19. http://dx.doi.org/10.1080/1359813022013227l

Reilly, J.M., Trial, J., Piver, D., & Schaff, P. (2012). Using theatre to increase empathy training in medical students. *Journal for Learning through Arts, 8*(1), 1–8.

Rodenhauser, P., Strickland, M.A., & Gambala, C.T. (2004, Summer). Arts-related activities across U.S. medical schools: a follow-up study. *Teaching and Learning in Medicine: An International Journal, 16*(3), 233–239. http://dx.doi.org/10.1207/s15328015tlm1603_2 Medline:15388377

5

Reader's Theatre and Sharing the Experience of Caregiving

Home Is Where the Heart Is

Maura McIntyre

This paper draws from qualitative research that seeks to provide a window into the functioning of the dynamic social environment of a publicly funded nursing home in a large Canadian urban centre; to better understand how staff contribute, beyond role definition or job description, to the residential environment as a home-like setting; and to gain insights into the complex interaction between individuals' personal and professional commitment to caregiving. I consider how, in the institutional context of the nursing home, these concepts are brought to life and made real through staff practices. I deconstruct the concept of homemaking and reinvent the meaning and significance of homemaking as care. Using reader's theatre as a presentation format, I discuss the qualities of the form and invite the reader to experience home *and* care *as psychological constructs through storied text and in-role performance.*

Research as Advocacy Work

My broad intention—making nursing homes and the people who live and work in them more accessible, more understandable and more inviting to family caregivers and the general public—identifies my research as advocacy work. My research is specifically about staff: who they are as people and what they can teach us about the place and people of nursing homes. In celebrating nursing-home workers as people, I also promote the act of giving care as a worthy activity. To render my research results best and to remain congruent with my commitment to accessibility, I use reader's theatre as a "data display strategy" and presentation form (Donmoyer & Donmoyer, 2008). *Home is where the heart is: A reader's theatre* involves a dramatic rendering of research results and as such is part of the growing genre of performance ethnography (Saldaña, 2008; Conquergood, 1991; McCall, 2000; Gray & Sinding, 2002).

Reader's Theatre

Within arts-informed research methodologies, reader's theatre is considered "relatively conservative" because data-collection methods do not typically involve processes related to the arts but rather rely on the traditional data-gathering techniques of in-depth interviews and participant observation (Donmoyer & Donmoyer, 2008, p. 210). Reader's theatre is also relatively straightforward to present. In this case the reader's theatre performance required no props, lighting or costumes, no time-consuming memorization of lines, rehearsal or preparation. The organizer invited audience members to participate on the spot, and volunteers were given reading parts or a script that they held and read. A reader's theatre can also be rehearsed in advance or even performed by professional actors to enhance the quality of presentation.

Despite the contrived nature of the prepared script, reader's theatre is thrilling because it is live. But while it invites an emotional response, reader's theatre also requires members of the audience to think. Instead of sitting back and riding through a story arc from beginning to end, in reader's theatre the themes and ideas presented display a diversity of perspectives. Integrating emotion with intellect, reader's theatre energizes the audience and provokes discussion about the issues and questions raised in the content of the work.

I chose reader's theatre as a presentation form for a variety of reasons. It allowed me to remain true to the storied nature of what I had been told as a researcher and to use everyday, ordinary language. I wanted to honour the complexity and the diversity of the stories in the retelling, and I wanted to create, through artistic form, the type of reflective conversation so many staff said they needed to have. The reader's theatre format carries content and is able to render an important aspect of my research results experientially.

Research Context and Method

The research is broadly qualitative and is situated more specifically within a community-centred, arts-informed life-history framework (McIntyre & Cole, 2008; McIntyre, 2000; Eisner, 1993). It was conducted in a publicly funded and operated 456-bed nursing home in a large urban centre in Canada. One specific objective, which is the focus of *Home is where the heart is*, was to better understand how individual staff contribute, beyond role definition or job description, to the environment as a home-like setting.

Unit-based staff who participated included personnel from housekeeping (heavy equipment and light duty), nursing (personal-care aides, nurse manager, charge nurses), recreation (recreational assistant), food service (server staff) and social work (social worker). Home-wide staff who participated included the home administrator, the director of nursing, the manager of programs and services, two complementary-care assistants (aromatherapy/therapeutic touch and music therapy), an occupational therapist, the spiritual and religious care coordinator, the supervisor of staff education and development, a psycho-geriatric consultant and a resident food-service supervisor. In total I conducted 15 interviews.

My data-collection methods included in-depth interviews with this diversity of personnel, the examination of pertinent institutional and personal artifacts and observations in context while spending time on the floor as a mealtime-assistance volunteer. Interview questions were open ended. Questions were clustered around three main areas: work profile, questions relating to beliefs about dementia and long-term care, and questions relating to personal life and experience.

Listening to the stories staff had to tell was an emotional experience. In conversation after conversation I was moved by how much of themselves staff put into their efforts to connect with residents. Such attentive and loving care seemed to require an analytical framework where this emotional quality could be preserved. Tom Kitwood's (1997) model of person-centred care, which describes the main psychological needs of a person with dementia as attachment, identity, occupation, comfort and inclusion, with love overarching all, provided just this framework. I proceeded with data analysis guided by this model and clustered emergent themes (such as food) according to a framing question (see below). In constructing the reader's theatre script I used attachment, identity, occupation, comfort and inclusion as themes within an organizing device for illumination as to how loving care was provided.

Institutional Care and the Meaning of Home

I begin by exploring *care* and *home* as separate concepts and mapping the terrain of their intersection through academic theory and everyday discourse. Since these two words peppered every interview with staff, deconstructing the complexity of the various meanings associated with them provides a useful context when I consider the issues staff raised. I consider how, in the institutional context of the nursing home, these concepts are made real through the practices of staff. I touch on the points of congruence and tension between individual staff members' values and beliefs about care and the structures in which they work by exploring the general question, *How do institutional structures support or constrain staff efforts to give care and make home?*

In exploring how individual staff members make home in the institution, I deconstruct *homemaking* and reinvent the meaning and significance of homemaking as care. I invite the reader to experience *home* and *care* as psychological constructs through storied text and in-role performance. Direct quotations from staff and sections of storied text (taken and extrapolated from interview data) appear in italics. In the live presentation of this paper these parts are given to audience members to read aloud in a reader's theatre presentation format. (I hold numbered cards up and people chime in when it is their turn.) I function as the host or narrator reading the background text (non-italicized).

When audience members speak the words as staff, they experience the narrative and the complexities of nursing-home life. By joining in and celebrating the work of caregiving and honouring the capacity to care, we broaden and extend the community supporting people living with dementia. This process of deconstructing practices of homemaking through alternative forms allows the work to inform and educate diverse audiences—including the general public, family caregivers and academics alike—about the people who work in nursing homes and the complexity of making home in the institution.

Notions of House and Home

In everyday discourse our notions of *home* and its significance as a social and psychological construct pepper our conversation. When we use the term *housewife*, or the somewhat less politically outdated term *homemaker*, we delineate occupation, identity and gender. On the other hand, do we imagine someone described as a *homebody* as male or female, young or old, vaguely anti-social or grounded and calm? And what is implied when a place is described as *homey* or a person is seen as *homely?* We extend hospitality and warmth by inviting guests *to make themselves at home.* We refer to feelings of comfort and connection by distinguishing between feeling *at home* or *not at home.* A *home away from home* comes close to satisfying our yearning for belonging. Conversely, the euphemism *there's no one home* suggests a kind of psychological vacantness. In keeping with this construction, the sense of stigma surrounding a *homeless person* suggests that the individual lacks much more than a fixed address.

The word *house,* on the other hand, tends to refer less to feelings and qualities of experience and more to physical setting. Lawless and Pietropaulo (2002) describe "house as the structural form of a site that exists in real time and space and that is a relatively stable entity" (p. 2). Our house is the roof over our head at any given time. It is the floorboards, the apartment, the dorm room, the address. Our sense of home, on the other hand, "usually can be, but not always is, contained or enclosed by a house" (p. 2). A home is in process; it is fluid, not fixed; it can exist in a garden, in a person or in a house; it involves coming and going and returning home once again: "Home represents an ideal place to experience our sense of intimacy" (Lawless & Pietropaulo, 2002, p. xi). We make and remake home, thus imbuing our notions of home with significance and meaning.

Marcus (1995) further distinguishes between the concepts of house and home. She suggests we use *house* as a "symbol of our place in society" (p. 12). Buying a house is a rite of passage associated with settling down, domesticity and a certain level of prosperity. How we give place meaning, Marcus suggests, comes from the interplay of our unconscious and conscious selves. While our houses contain representations of conscious self-expression—that is, they convey identity and say who we are through choice of colour, objects and furniture—our homes also contain expressions of the self that are unconscious. She suggests that the "soul-seeds" of feeling rooted in place have to do with emotional connection and are sown during the "innocent openness" of early childhood (Marcus, 1995, p. 254). Later in life, when we feel deeply "at home" we are reconnecting with that soul-nurturing place where we experience emotional attachment. Home is thus constructed as "a symbol of psychic wholeness" (Jung, 1969 in Marcus, 1995, p. xvi).

In keeping with this distinction between house and home, I consider efforts that have to do with improving the physical plan of a place—things like wallpaper, knick-knacks and furniture—to be quite different from acts of care made by people. While these "home improvements" are not without significance—and in the nursing-home environment they affect the well-being of staff, residents and visitors alike—their impact on the sense of home of the place pales in comparison to the impact of the presence of the people in that place.

From the script:

> *I think that what makes it a home first and foremost is the caring attitude of the staff. They treat residents as though they're part of their own family. They do for them what they would do for their own family member and although the environment has a lot to do with it, you can go into a nursing home that has the ensuite washrooms and everything else, but it can feel very, very, cold.* (McIntyre, 2005)

As with our houses, a nursing home can perpetually renovate and decorate, yet the place may feel no more like a home than when the initiative to make "home improvements" began. As Bachelard (1958) describes, our need for home cannot be completely satisfied through cosmetic improvements because the "images of protected intimacy" of which notions of home are made resonant on a much deeper level (p. 6). Throughout our lives "we comfort ourselves by reliving memories of protection" that we overlay with images of home (p. 6).

Notions of Care and Love

Even a surface reading of everyday talk reveals the images of care and love embedded in our notions of home. Conversely, an exploration of the qualities of love and care reveals their close relationship to our notions of home. Even when people have had no actual experience of a "loving home," powerful images of an ideal home remain throughout the lifespan (Gubrium, 1993, 1976). When nursing home residents repeat the refrain "I want to go home" or when people suffering from dementia engage in so-called exit-seeking behaviour, they likely long for this psychological home, an ideal separate from time and space.

In *The philosophy of existentialism* (1956), Gabriel Marcel characterizes love and care together as "creative fidelity," "attentive listening" and "meaningful solidarity." Tom Kitwood (1997) names love as the main psychological need of people with dementia. In Kitwood's model of person-centred care, love is active: love is as love does. Loving care brings the person with dementia opportunities for attachment, identity, inclusion, occupation and comfort (Kitwood, 1997). The boundaries of these needs overlap and combine, and even in people who are independent and well, Kitwood points out, they are not necessarily in evidence most of the time (Kitwood, 1997). The meeting of even one of these needs, however, can advance the fulfillment of another.

Person-Centred Loving Care

Attachment is a universal human need that can become more pronounced in people with dementia because they frequently find the familiar strange. Feelings of attachment are at the root of our capacity to feel "at home."

2.

We make sure that we have lots of magazines available, open shelves, things residents can pick up. It doesn't matter that it disappears, the staff can pick it up at some other point and bring it back. We have hats, things for the men, dolls, stuffed animals, purses, things that were familiar. (McIntyre, 2005)

Attachment is reciprocal.

3.

I feel very much alive when I am able to cry when a resident dies. I recognize that that's a healthy place to be in. I remember once, not too long ago, a resident passing away and I started crying and I think if the charge nurse cries it almost gives other people on the team permission to feel, and I think as long as you're feeling, you're living fully. I think the more closed we become, the more emotionally shut down we are. Ultimately that's not a healthy or an empathetic place for caregivers to be. It's better to stay close to your emotions.

1(a).

For a while there, like the first, I guess, 17 years ... what I found really difficult about my work ... was the death. The anticipation of death is constant. I took it very personally because every resident I did care about. I started visiting people in the hospital that were sick. And so, every day, I would go and visit people that were sick and go to funerals of people that died and after a while I was getting up at eight o'clock going to the hospitals, then going to funerals and then going to work. I did this for a couple of months but then I said too much, I've got to stop this. I just packed it in and I said I'll go in and do my time, listen to stories and when they're gone I'll remember the good stuff. You know when you're there emotionally ... and you're going to see death almost every week, so if you wait for it or you contemplate it or you dwell on it, it will just eat you up. (McIntyre, 2005)

The need to feel occupied in a way that is consistent with individual ability also begins very early in life and persists across the lifespan. Occupation, however, should not be confused with "busy work." Occupation is tied to agency, and for people with dementia, agency is as linked to self-esteem as it is to people who are well (Kitwood, 1997).

4.

We're getting residents involved now in washing clothes and ironing. That's why the breakfast club is so popular, it's a normalizing environment. I bought griddles and coffee percolators because we want them to smell the coffee perking and that kind of thing. We have a breadmaker as well. The residents measure out all the ingredients to make the bread ... they're part of the whole thing and they get to eat the bread afterwards when it's ready. (McIntyre, 2005)

The human need for inclusion, to feel a part of the social group, is also necessary for survival.

5.

Often I notice people, I'm singing a song, an old familiar song, and someone with severe dementia might be breathing at the right time. They're not actually singing, they might be vocalizing a little, but they're breathing when I'm breathing! I've had some families who weren't visiting relatives anymore because it's too painful for them, and then it's like, "Oh, you have them in a group and they're getting all this attention." And they get involved again almost because the facility is treating this person like a person still, you know, like a deserving, worthy, person. (McIntyre, 2005)

For people with dementia, the awareness that they are different, and the realities of the social stigma associated with their condition, can lead to feelings of profound isolation and exclusion.

6.

We're all required to do one evening every two weeks. I enjoy going up to the floor and seeing residents in the evening. It's quiet. The isolation that they feel is so obvious. I like being able to, kind of, you know, come into that. (McIntyre, 2005)

Individualized care plans for people with dementia often overlook social history and the person's current needs for inclusion (Kitwood, 1997).

7.

I think the environment has a lot to do with it, but it's really how you make the environment work for the residents, how you make them feel they're at home, they're not confined to certain areas, you know, don't cross over this line. They're free to come and go as they please, to go wherever they like to go, participate in whatever they like to participate in. They're encouraged to participate. (McIntyre, 2005)

On the other hand, individual care plans have helped caregivers to address the ongoing need of people with dementia to experience identity. Understanding a person's history and recognizing the capacity for empathy are the main ways we acknowledge each other as people and confer identity.

8.

The more we share information about who residents are, the more we share what works. The secret of long-term care boils down to what works for Mary, and everybody on the team needs to know what works for Mary and what doesn't. And if we haven't shared that information with them, I don't think we're doing our job. It takes you so long to get that information. And whether you get it from direct conversation with a family member or whether you intuitively stumble across it, it's wisdom. It helps develop caring and empathy in caregivers. (McIntyre, 2005)

Comfort "carries meanings of tenderness, closeness, the soothing of pain and sorrow, the calming of anxiety, [and] the feeling of security which comes from being close to another" (Kitwood, 1997, p. 81). The close association between being comforted and feeling comfortable and at home is implicit.

9.

> I'm a complementary-care assistant, which means basically I do aromatherapy, massage and therapeutic touch. One of the really good things about my job is that it's pretty open. I have a basin of hot water and I'll put in some essential oils like lemon or something kind of refreshing. Usually the room is small enough that the essential oil can scent the room. They always have the TV on, but I can never tell how many people are actually watching it. So I put in a video of a fish tank with just, just fish swimming around. It's a nice soothing background in the room. So I put in that, I put on some nice relaxing music, and then I usually go around with the face cloth and I dip it in the water and give it to people. And they're great. Like there was one man in particular he washes his whole face and scrubs his neck and when he gives it back to me, he's all refreshed ... (McIntyre, 2005)

Kitwood (1997) suggests that loving care is expressed through "the sensitive meeting of this cluster of needs" and the personhood of an individual with dementia is maintained (p. 84). He distinguishes between "person-centered care," which foregrounds the holistic needs of a person with dementia, and "task-centered care," which focuses less on the person and more on particular tasks (such as bathing or changing) that need to be accomplished (Kitwood, 1997).

10.

> Not resident-focused is someone who is stuck, who thinks the most important thing is sticking to routines. "These are the absolute routines. This is what we do. Your bath day is on Tuesday because there are far too many people getting bathed on Monday. No, we bathe everybody in the morning, evening staff are far too busy to be bathing, you know that." And you can't be like that. You have to find out what's important to those individuals. You have to have a unit that supports residents who want to sleep in, and if they do sleep in, how are you going to get them something to eat before lunch. You can make all of these things work, you just have to have the will to do it. Or you can stick to the rules. Sticking to the rules means you may run a very efficient unit but it's a cold unit where the residents are a product, not people. (McIntyre, 2005)

Person-centred caring requires a degree of personal presence or, to use Nel Noddings' (1984) term, "engrossment" on the part of the one caring (p. 19). The one caring needs to place the person he/she is caring for in the centre of his/her sights, both literally and emotionally, to convey care fully. The "motivational displacement" required to accomplish this degree of presence is usually contrary to staff job descriptions that are task centred rather than person centred (Noddings, 1984, p. 25). Job descriptions tend to describe what the staff person must do, not how it would be helpful for them to be.

9(a).

I'm lucky because it's a part of my job to actually go in and sit down with the residents, and maybe have a little one to one interaction. Or you know just hold their hand ... you know this is what I'm actually supposed to be doing. Whereas I know a lot of the personal care assistants or nurses they might not have time to do that. (McIntyre, 2005)

For people with dementia, the process of making a nursing home feel like home is not characterized by a discrete period of adjustment. Indeed, Shield (1988) suggests that even cognitively intact residents never really "settle in" because nursing home life is an "endless transition" between adult life in the community and death to come (p. 184). The very notion of settling in is an illusion in the "liminality" that is the reality of nursing-home life (Shield, 1988).

A more hopeful vision places opportunities to make home in the hands of people who give care. For people with dementia, life is an ongoing process of trying to get their psychological needs met in the face of failing mental powers. People with dementia are particularly vulnerable to feeling homeless. Simply put, feeling less sure of who we are, or of where we belong, makes the longing for home both more pronounced and more profound. Unfortunately, initiatives such as "wandering," "hoarding" or "hovering" that people with dementia take to express these needs are often seen as symptoms or pathology. When individual staff persons are able to see beyond these behaviours to the human need being expressed, person-centred care is provided. Care that addresses the fulfillment of the main psychological needs of people with dementia invokes the presence of home, no matter where that caring occurs. Well or ill, when we feel deeply at home, our psychological needs are in some important way being met.

11.

It starts with the nurse manager on the floor and the tone that that individual sets and the partnership that they have with the recreational staff, housekeeping staff, rehab, foodservice, everyone. All the other partners that are part of the team. It's the texture of those relationships. If that person is really inclusive and resident-focused and has the residents' best interests at heart ... it will all come together. (McIntyre, 2005)

Ultimately the people are the place or, as Bachelard (1958) poetically explains, "all really inhabited space bears the essence of the notion of home" (p. 5). While the sheer numbers of people at nursing homes challenge traditional notions of intimacy and of home, person-centred care nurtures the closeness and connection of an ideal home.

12.

Some of them don't know me by name but they'll call me "the food lady." I'm "the food lady" or "the food nurse." Officially I'm one of three resident food service supervisors in this home. I'm responsible for two hundred residents.

I like trying to do things that make the day a little easier for the resident. A cheese sandwich with jam instead of tuna or ham—it's a small thing, but if Mr. Sanchez likes cheese and jam, it means something. I try and keep it simple. I say: "Let's eat!" I show them the chicken. I show them the cannelloni. It's all presentation ... even people who still know, they want to see what food they're choosing.

The social dynamics of eating, they're just as important as the actual meal itself. Because if they're not happy with who they're sitting with, they're not eating. We have two ladies that sit together and they don't really want anyone to sit with anyone else, and let me tell you they make that clear. Another lady, who's over 100, she wants a conversation. Anybody who can't feed themselves or speak up for themselves, she doesn't want to sit with. I think she's 106 now.

11(a).

How can you feed thirteen residents with four staff in half and hour? It's very difficult for staff, especially since they want to do a good job. Paperwork is different. You can put it aside, or take it home and do it. But with resident care, you can't. Generally staff want to provide the quality of care that they're expected to, and they find that they just can't keep up ... That brings up lots of hard feelings.

12(a).

These days people are coming in sicker ... more progressed with disease. You see them in a later stage of life than when they were baking the cakes and doing the birthday parties and dancing in the dining room. It's important to find out what the individual needs and what the group at each table wants. Do they prefer to have tea before the meal or afterwards? Are there other rituals around eating—like prayer—that we can help with? Are there couples who want to sit, the two together, off to the side, alone?

Sometimes family members have ideas about what we can do ... Their father will only eat their mother's cooking. Well, we can't cook the same way your mother did in this kitchen. And even if I wanted to cook in my own kitchen I couldn't cook like your mother did. But if you want to bring the food in ... we can accommodate that. We'll store it, we'll heat it up, and we'll serve it the best we can.

I grew up in a small town, about 6000 people, on a dairy farm. I did a lot of manual work when I was young. It was a real family farm, we worked together, my parents were always home. I'm no city slicker.

I don't like to cook or anything. I can cook a decent meal but I'm not going to make an elaborate meal for anybody, right?

13.

I just have to tell you this story. On the sixth floor there are a large number of Portuguese residents and I have Portuguese recreation staff and there are Portuguese housekeeping staff—in fact they are the ones that actually point out certain needs of the residents. For example, my rec staff said to me, "You know the Portuguese observe this Portuguese day of grace and I'd really like to do something with it." So I said, "Well, tell me what it is." She replied, "It's almost a special religious type celebration, once a year." And I said, "So what would we be doing? I need the visual." And she said, "We can do a service in the worship centre. There would be a Portuguese priest that could come in and do the service and then we'll have this dinner in the auditorium." I said, "Okay, so who is providing this dinner? How are we doing this dinner?" And it was just really classic, but at first I thought, oh gosh, I don't know that I can do this. She said, "Don't worry, just leave it to me and I'm going to go out in the community and I'm going to get donations for this, that, and the other and you don't have to worry." And I'm thinking, oh, this sounds huge, like how can you do this? Anyway, I trust my staff and I know she does an excellent job and she went out into the community and she had this whole entourage of church volunteers come in from a particular church. They brought all their huge pans from the church kitchen. Out here I had, I can't tell you, how many chickens and how many bags of carrots and potatoes, and the chopping and everything that was going on. I just sat here saying, "I don't know how this is going to end up."

But they cooked up all this stuff, and the auditorium when I went in there was absolutely amazing. They had transformed it into the Azores. They had the video going. They had all their lace. They had traditional costumes. They had ... the entire auditorium was Portuguese. It was just amazing. The room was packed. We had a hundred, and I don't know, twenty people and I said, how do we have 120 people, we only have I don't know, 40 Portuguese residents or whatever, but we had 120 people in this room. All there for dinner, the auction was going on, they raised money for the floor. Everybody had a great time. And then it became an annual event.

12(b).

That *is* quite a story.

Anyhow, you know how I said I'm no city slicker? Well, sometimes I do go to Starbucks for a treat. I'm no regular. But every few months it's Saturday and I've been shopping and I do enjoy a warm beverage around four o'clock. Maybe a little sweet too. So I step into Starbucks and I'm immediately overtaken with all the delicious smells, and the colours of the walls, so I just sort of stand there staring at the menu for a while. Toffee Nut Late, Vanilla Latte, Caramel Machiato, White Chocolate Mocha … I just roll the names around in my mouth … they all sound so plumped up and fluffy.

After a while I realize that I'm still just sort of standing there my eyes slightly closed, head tilted back, loving the smells … and the chipper server guy behind the counter has looked at me again and this time his eyebrow is a bit raised.

So I figure I better bear down on the menu. Scanning the board I'm looking for one of those new sweet black teas that's cooked up with spices. Chai. It's called chai. But is it tazo hot tea, or tazo chai that I like?

Further down I notice another whole tea section with tazo citrus, tazo berry and tazo chai crème. A line is starting to form so I don't take the time to ask the server guy the difference between tazo and tea, chai and tazo chai. I order a grande tazo chai crème … which I know from experience is the medium size, and start rummaging around in my wallet, trying to quickly produce the $4.15, oh, but with tax it will be what? $4.50 or so.

Off to the side now I watch the server gal artfully construct my beverage. I get mesmerized again by all the pouring and measuring, and testing of temperatures. And I start to think about all the things we do to try and keep the residents' food hot, coming all that way from the kitchen in the basement to the floors. The new steam tables we got on the units, the meetings we had trying to tighten up the system between the elevator porter and the servery staff, the hot holding carts … and still it's not perfect. Three meals a day, with a choice between two entrees at each meal in five different textures: regular, mince, purees, dental soft, and chopped. Do people have any idea how complex it is, providing food for older people—people who are losing their teeth and their capacity to swallow? The special diets for health—lactose intolerant, low sodium, high calorie, and low spice. Snacks three times a day—a sandwich or some digestive cookies, tea or juice or maybe a glass of milk. The different tastes and preferences, the religious restrictions like pork and special foods for holidays. Suddenly Starbucks seems simple.

I laugh out loud when I realize that what I've paid—$4.65 with tax, for my grande tazo chai crème—my Saturday after shopping treat, is 16 cents more than our per day resident food budget. Yeah, that's right—three meals a day, with a choice between two entrees at each meal in five different textures: regular, mince, puree, dental soft, and chopped. Plus snacks with a beverage at 10:00, at 2:00 and before bed at 8:00. Plus tea and cookies during the night for the wanderers. All that for $4.49 per resident per day. It's gone up 23 cents since 1993. Ten years and an increase in 23 cents per day per person. How much do you figure Starbucks has put up their prices in ten years?

1(b).

A few years back during one of those restructurings, it looked like the place was going to go private, sold off … bought up … And that's pretty scary because you think these people are going to come in and they want to make a profit so they don't want all the stuff you do, basically they don't care what your philosophy is, just do the work, cut costs, don't use too many linens. Lots of paperwork with being public, but trust me, it's a whole lot better than care for profit. (McIntyre, 2005)

Caring to Make Home

Exploring our notions of care and home begins to reveal the complexity of the term *nursing home.* The name itself carries the tension of conflicting expectations. A site of medical practice overlaid with images of protection, comfort and intimacy: what might that look like? And how should we expect that place to feel? Do we somehow equate institutionalization with homelessness? And further, in caring for a loved one with dementia at home, is the effort to resist institutionalization also an effort to resist an additional stigma—that of homelessness? Is it surprising that research shows that the sense of loss associated with placing a loved one in long-term care, combined with negative preconceptions about nursing homes in general, often leads to a disjuncture between family expectations and the actual care provided (Krause, Grant & Long, 1999; Foner, 1995)?

14.

One of our biggest challenges is trying to get families engaged, to be part of the process, and breaking down their initial fear and hostility. It's a big, big, place and initially I think people are frightened and acting out of fear. They react in anger and sometimes say things that are really inappropriate to staff. I've been in the cafeteria and overheard people talking as though none of us are there, you know, "What kind of dump is this? Look at the crap they're serving." How do you deal with that? Should I walk up and say, "Hi. I'm the administrator. Do you want to come and talk to me?" They don't really want to talk. Some folks just want to make a scene. (McIntyre, 2005)

Epilogue

Each time I present my research as a reader's theatre (in public libraries, at academic conferences and at forums of health care workers), a space is provided to recognize and honour the people who care for people living with dementia and to consider the realities and possibilities of nursing-home life. I always name and make explicit the tribute aspect of my work—in academic presentations and public venues alike. No one ever balks. People are always respectful of my intentions. Indeed, they are quick to volunteer as readers. Reading aloud in a group brings out the very best in people. They speak with spirit, from the heart.

When people honour my research participants and my writing with their voices and speak from the position of nursing-home workers, they make audible voices that are rarely widely heard. As the readers come together in what could be described as a political act, the atmosphere reverberates with a feeling of communion by the time the last voice is heard. A palette of tones resonates through the room. The experience begins to feel like more than the sum of its parts. Hope emerges.

In light of the current and projected need for institutional care, opportunities to create hope and inspiration to give care are critical. Simply put, we will be needing a new generation of people who care to make home.

NOTE

This article was originally published in CCAHTE (*Canadian Creative Arts in Health, Training and Education Journal*) (7) January 20, 2009.

REFERENCES

Bachelard, G. (1958). *The poetics of space.* Boston, Mass: Beacon Press.

Conquergood, D. (1991). Rethinking ethnography: Towards a critical cultural politics. *Communication Monographs, 58*(2), 179–194. http://dx.doi.org/10.1080/03637759109376222

Donmoyer, R., & Donmoyer, J.Y. (2008). Readers' theatre as a data display strategy. In J.G. Knowles & A.L. Cole (Eds.), *Handbook of the arts in qualitative research: Perspectives, methodologies, examples, and issues* (pp. 209–224). Thousand Oaks, CA: Sage. http://dx.doi.org/10.4135/9781452226545.n18

Eisner, E.W. (1993). Forms of understanding and the future of educational research. *Educational Researcher, 22*(7), 5–11. http://dx.doi.org/10.3102/0013189X022007005

Foner, N. (1995). Relatives as trouble: Nursing home aides and patients' families. In J. Henderson & M. Vesperi (Eds.), *The culture of long term care: Nursing home ethnography* (pp. 165–178). Westport, CT: Bergin & Garvey.

Gray, R., & Sinding, C. (2002). *Standing Ovation: Performing social science research about cancer.* Walnut Creek, CA: AltaMira Press.

Gubrium, J. (1976). *Living and dying at Murray Manor.* New York: St. Martin's Press.

Gubrium, J. (1993). *Speaking of life.* New York: Aldine de Gruyter, Inc.

Jung, C. (1969). *Memories, dreams, reflections.* London: Fontana Library.

Kitwood, T. (1997). *Dementia reconsidered: The person comes first.* London: Open University Press.

Krause, A., Grant, L., & Long, B. (1999). Sources of stress reported by daughters of nursing home residents. *Journal of Aging Studies, 13*(3), 349–364. http://dx.doi.org/10.1016/S0890-4065(99)80101-7

Lawless, C., & Pietropaulo, V. (2002). *Making home in Havana.* New Brunswick, NJ: Rutgers University Press.

Marcel, G. (1956). *The philosophy of existentialism.* New York: The Citadel Press.

Marcus, C. (1995). *House as a mirror of self: Exploring the deeper meaning of home.* Berkeley, CA: Conari Press.

McCall, M. (2000). Performance ethnography: A brief history and some advice. In N.K. Denzin & Y.S. Lincoln (Eds.), *The handbook of qualitative research* (2nd ed., pp. 421–435). Thousand Oaks, CA: Sage.

McIntyre, M. (2000). *Garden as phenomenon, method and metaphor in the context of health care: An arts informed life history view.* Unpublished doctoral dissertation. Ontario Institute for Studies in Education at the University of Toronto, Toronto, Canada.

McIntyre, M. (2005). *RESPECT. A reader's theatre about people who care for people in nursing homes.* Halifax, NS: Backalong Books.

McIntyre, M., & Cole, A. (2008, Mar). Love stories about caregiving and Alzheimer's disease: a performative methodology. *Journal of Health Psychology, 13*(2), 213–225. http://dx.doi.org/10.1177/1359105307086701 Medline:18375627

Noddings, N. (1984). *Caring: A feminine approach to ethics and moral education.* Berkeley, CA: University of California Press.

Saldaña, J. (2008). Ethnodrama and ethnotheatre. In J.G. Knowles & A.L. Cole (Eds.), *Handbook of the arts in qualitative research: Perspectives, methodologies, examples, and issues* (pp. 195–207). Thousand Oaks, CA: Sage. http://dx.doi.org/10.4135/9781452226545.n17

Shield, R. (1988). *Uneasy endings: Daily life in an American nursing home.* Ithaca, NY: Cornell University Press.

6

The Stanford Arts and Anesthesia Soiree

Performing to Create Community and Understand Anesthesiology

Craig Chen, MD, Natalya Hasan, MD,
Julie Good, MD, and Audrey Shafer, MD

We believe the arts and humanities are integral to medicine. In 2012, the *New England Journal of Medicine* published an article by David Watts, "Cure for the common cold," which challenges medical educators to revolutionize the teaching of bedside manners and compassionate care. "A dose of literature," he writes, "has resonance for the practice of medicine." Watts argues that experiencing, discussing and engaging with the humanities are more effective in teaching the art of medicine than lectures and textbooks.

Recognizing that incorporating the arts and humanities into the culture of our large academic anesthesia department might improve wellness for residents and prevent physician burnout, we sought to create a deeper sense of community by highlighting department members' talents. An organizing committee made up of faculty, staff, an emeritus physician, a fellow and residents created an event titled the Stanford Arts and Anesthesia Soiree and encouraged members of the department and their families to share artistic and creative works. Presentations included filmmaking, writing, visual art, musical and dance performances and crafts. While some submissions reflected on patient interactions, we also encouraged non-medical art.

This program was much more than a social gathering. Rather, it was an energizing, innovative and inspiring space for health care professionals to connect outside the world of medicine. Our intent was to engage each other through the arts in a non-medical setting, to stimulate humanistic discussion about anesthesia and to break down academic hierarchies. We wanted to get to know our colleagues as multi-dimensional people and to encourage them to foster interests that make them unique. We intermixed performances by attending physicians, residents, alumni, certified registered nurse anesthetists, anesthesia technicians, research faculty and staff, breaking down barriers created by our professional roles.

One of the best-received performances was an anesthesia technician singing rhythm and blues accompanied by an anesthesia resident on piano. This collaboration between an allied healthcare worker and a physician in training showed how their mutual love for music could transcend professional roles to create a beautiful, moving performance. The event also enabled department members to include family members as participants. For example, we welcomed a mother-and-son trumpet duet, a family string quartet and origami created by children of a faculty member.

The Stanford Arts and Anesthesia Soiree helped us see our colleagues in a different light, sharing identities defined by more than

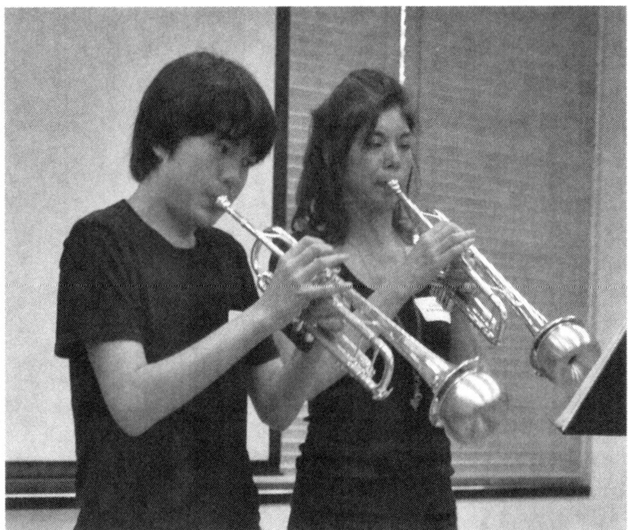

Figure 6.1 Dr. Louise Furukawa, pediatric anesthesiologist, accompanies her son Jordan in a jazz duet at the Arts and Anesthesia Soiree.

profession. One anesthesiologist, for example, read two poems about his emotional turmoil resulting from the Syrian civil war and its effects on his family. Listening, we were moved by his humanity and impressed by his courage. As we rose in a standing ovation, we came together as a community, enriched by the experience.

As poets explored themes such as the responsibility of caring for a patient under anesthesia, the development of trust with one's patients and rituals in the operating room, our non-medical family and colleagues gained greater insight into our daily emotions, challenges, achievements and satisfactions. At the reception after the performances, we overheard comments like, "I had no idea how stressful my husband's job is on a daily basis." Administrative staff within the department expressed that they learned more about the physician's experience from the soiree. One of the authors of this paper found that writing poetry for the soiree motivated him to reflect on and reinterpret the experience of delivering anesthesia. In the poem "Song," he asks, "Where is that limit beyond which the body no longer sings/ but cries out, beyond which we, with all our draughts and devices and guilement/cannot rescue the body from the enchanted sleep we devise and the sleep it craves?"

Song

Words nestle into the cadence of the heart,
the body's metronome. Time and sustenance marked
in this alien landscape, its orbiting moons gathering light
in handfuls and dispersing it on the body,
a body alien, framed in blue, rubbed deep brown
awaiting the brave and foreign to part its skin.

The heart knows, accelerando!
the anesthetized body's tongue. Even in this state
the heart has reasons that reason knows not.
Even in this state, the body sings
We are interpreters of language.
Anesthesia is a fascination with the surrender of body,
muting before interrogation, a reversal
of things natural, a conscientious poisoning.

The more we inhale those fumes,
the more we realize it is as much a snare
for the recipient as the giver, that as we
tame more and more of the wild,
we become more ambitious
in some quest to cure human ailment.

Where is that border? Where is that limit
beyond which the body no longer sings
but cries out, beyond which we, with all
our draughts and devices and guilement
cannot rescue the body from
the enchanted sleep we devise
and the sleep it craves?

—Craig Chen

In a field traditionally viewed as technical and impersonal, the arts and humanities allow us to share and educate others about the physician's experience as well as reflect on our own feelings, insecurities and curiosities. As physician burnout involves emotional exhaustion, depersonalization and a sense of low personal accomplishment (Shanafelt, Sloan & Habermann, 2003), the Stanford Arts and Anesthesia Soiree addressed well-being by engaging the community with discussion about the stresses of clinical care and the memorable patients we see, as well as exploring the reasons why we entered the field of medicine.

The Anesthesiologist Sees Pink

Moonrise in a curved pink sky
a perfect fingernail for my oximeter.

A screen of pink pink pink
obliterates the shoehorn edge of epiglottis:
fiber optic frustration.

Carbon dioxide pooches the umbilical hernia,
a cupola between worlds,
above a pink peritoneal dome.

Spectra of effluvia:
ascites the color of birchwood
urine blued by indigo carmine
flecks of gold in malachite bile
but one color demands intensive care—
the thin pink froth of pulmonary edema
flooding the accordion circuit.

Inside all of us, life blushes pink and moist
our passage till black and white hardens
dry gangrene, bleached bone.

Yet even as winter chills, there,
just beyond my porch,
November camellias bloom
pulsing pink.

—Audrey Shafer

Lefebvre (2012) has characterized resident burnout as a tension between personal and professional responsibilities. Many residents have nurtured arts activities throughout their formative years, passions that have adorned their resumes throughout their schooling and training, but rarely do they have time to pursue those activities during residency. One resident said that preparing for the evening motivated him to polish his piano playing and rediscover music he loved. When he played Edward Grieg's "Wedding Day in Troldhaugen," the room was astonished by his manual dexterity and lyrical interpretation of the music.

A case study by Sullivan, Bucholz, Yeo, Roman, Bell, and Sosa (2012) suggests social interaction between attending physicians and residents improves residents' satisfaction and support networks. One goal of the Stanford Arts and Anesthesia Soiree was to enrich our sense of connection and community. During the reception, friends, family, residents and attending physicians discussed the experience of artwork openly in a forum free of academic hierarchies. The innovative, inspiring and energetic space created by our event provided an opportunity to strengthen the well-being of our physicians, allied healthcare workers and staff.

The response to the event was overwhelming. We had 16 performances, 24 artists with works on display and more than 130 attendees. We were surprised by the diversity of submissions, which included film, poetry and prose, classical and jazz music, choral performance, Chinese martial arts and ballroom dance. On display were paintings, photographs, origami, knitting, culinary arts, sewing and poetry.

Compassionate care and humane medicine are "less accessible to science than to art" and involve an experience that "is not primarily intellectual but emotional" (Watts, 2012). With the Stanford Arts and Anesthesia Soiree, we created a forum in which residents and staff nurtured the ideals, values and emotions and the creativity that motivated us to go into medicine in the first place. It is a space that rarely arises in the technical and scientific day-to-day practice of medicine. Ultimately, we created this initiative to celebrate the artistic, musical and emotional depth of the department, leading to a more coherent sense of community and a deeper understanding about anesthesiology. The arts and humanities remind us anesthesia is far more than merely medications and procedures.

REFERENCES

Lefebvre, D.C. (2012, May). Perspective: Resident physician wellness: a new hope. *Academic Medicine, 87*(5), 598–602. http://dx.doi.org/10.1097/ACM.0b013e31824d47ff Medline:22450179

Shanafelt, T.D., Sloan, J.A., & Habermann, T.M. (2003, Apr 15). The well-being of physicians. *American Journal of Medicine, 114*(6), 513–519. http://dx.doi.org/10.1016/S0002-9343(03)00117-7 Medline:12727590

Sullivan, M.C., Bucholz, E.M., Yeo, H., Roman, S.A., Bell, R.H., & Sosa, J.A. (2012, May). "Join the club": effect of resident and attending social interactions on overall satisfaction among 4390 general surgery residents. *Archives of Surgery, 147*(5), 408–414. http://dx.doi.org/10.1001/archsurg.2012.27 Medline:22785631

Watts, D. (2012, Sep 27). Cure for the common cold. *New England Journal of Medicine, 367*(13), 1184–1185. http://dx.doi.org/10.1056/NEJMp1209265 Medline:23013072

7

Art Practice and Bringing Emotions to Life in the Anatomy Lab

The Story of an Artist in Residence

Rachael Allen

The role of the artist is to challenge, change and provoke science.
—*J. McLachlan*

This article presents visual artwork and creative engagement from projects related to my practice as a fine artist and researcher working in the field of medical education and medical humanities and during my time as artist in residence (AIR) at university anatomy and clinical skills laboratories in the northeast of England. In this article I expand on the significance of medical students' expressing emotions, and how my arts practice supports this.

Project ANATOME emerged from my interest in opening "up" *(ana)* and "a cutting" *(tome)* of anatomic and medical pedagogy to create a dialogue among artistic methodologies, the sensory approach to anatomy and clinical studies and the undergraduate experience of medical education. The outcomes of the project take shape as artworks for exhibitions and events, academic papers for interdisciplinary conferences and symposia contributing to the field of medical humanities, published articles with artworks and creative activities engaging with undergraduate medicine.

Launched in 2011, the project is centred on the collaboration between me as artist and anatomy lecturer Dr. Gabrielle Finn at the School of Medicine, Pharmacy and Health, Durham University, with the support of the associate dean of the undergraduate medicine program, Professor John McLachlan. Both educators have widely published research on the application of art in undergraduate medicine and objective measures for medical-student professionalism. A major component of this project has been to assume the role of AIR within their medical department to observe teaching activity regularly and interact with undergraduate medical students and educators. In addition, I have established this role within two other institutions in the northeast of England: Newcastle Medical School, where undergraduate medicine is delivered through a partnership between Newcastle and Durham universities, and Northumbria University, where a Diploma of Higher Education in Medical Sciences is delivered in partnership with the first-year Postgraduate MD program offered by St. George's International School of Medicine, Grenada, West Indies.

Professor John McLachlan (2009) upholds the belief in the valuable influence of art in medical training, emphasizing, "... the role of the artist is to challenge, change and provoke science." At the heart of my artwork is the (re)presentation of the human body as the object of disease diagnosis and narrator of illness experience, drawing attention to modern bioethics and the (in)humane aspects of modern medicine. I also wish to share with medical students, educators and allied health professionals how interaction with a visual artist and the process of artmaking can help explore perceptions and offer ways to express emotions to promote the practice of humane medicine.

My practice enters the field of medical humanities by situating itself in one of its defining movements: the use of visual arts in educating medical pedagogy, medical practice and health care. The empirical research I perform within medical education and further afield highlights the problems, dilemmas and critical issues surrounding medicine today. Amalgamating these studies and AIR activity gives rise to visual art and literary work that offers new meanings and ways of conceiving humane medicine while exploring areas of bioethics, patient-and-doctor relationships, the history of medicine and anatomy, and illness phenomenology.

A growing number of programs in medical institutions worldwide encourage students to explore their emotions through self-reflection, art, journal writing, creative writing and group discussion (Coulehan, Williams, Landis & Naser, 1995; Marks, Bertman & Penney, 1997; Stewart and Charon, 2002; Rizzolo, 2002). It is on these grounds I endorse the application of AIR in medical education. Students must recognize, access, accept and express emotions throughout their journey to doctor-hood. Introspection is valuable, and when students talk about what they feel, they have the opportunity to learn about the diverse perspectives of their classmates and to reshape their attitudes toward patient care (Rizzolo, 2002). The artist can facilitate activities such as life drawing, self-reflective art-making and writing—accompanied by guided discussions—and can bring perspective to the complex environment where anatomy and medicine are taught.

In the following sections, I expand on the activity I undertook as AIR, the focus of Project ANATOME, the value of artistic intervention in medical education and the envisioned advances toward humane medicine. Featured activities include Specimen Life (Death) Drawing, Patient Study Module and Picturing Diagnosis, all of which draw inspiration from the field of medical humanities, illness phenomenology and the practice of narrative medicine. I also present examples of artworks and exhibitions that have derived from Project ANATOME and my AIR activity and suggest how they, too, can educate medical students and educators and contribute to the evolution of humane medicine.

AIR and Project ANATOME

As the AIR at a Durham, Newcastle and Northumbria University anatomy and clinical skills labs, I coordinate my observational research in line with taught classes, demonstrations, self-directed study and lectures. I witness a range of real and virtual anatomy teaching; prepared prosections of embalmed and plastinated specimens; anatomic models; living anatomy involving inspection, palpation, percussion and auscultation of live models or peer examination; medical imaging using X-ray, MRI and ultrasound; the Virtual Human Dissector; and body painting.

I focus on observing the way students interact with the embalmed and plastinated prosections: how they physically handle the specimens, their body language and facial expressions, the conversations that occur among peer groups and teaching staff, the conduct of all (living) present in the lab and the manner of interaction with all teaching materials. During this time, I also perform a degree of introspection as I, too, experience heightened emotions associated with the materiality of the bodies, the anomalous encounter of life and death in proximity and the provocation of ethical issues.

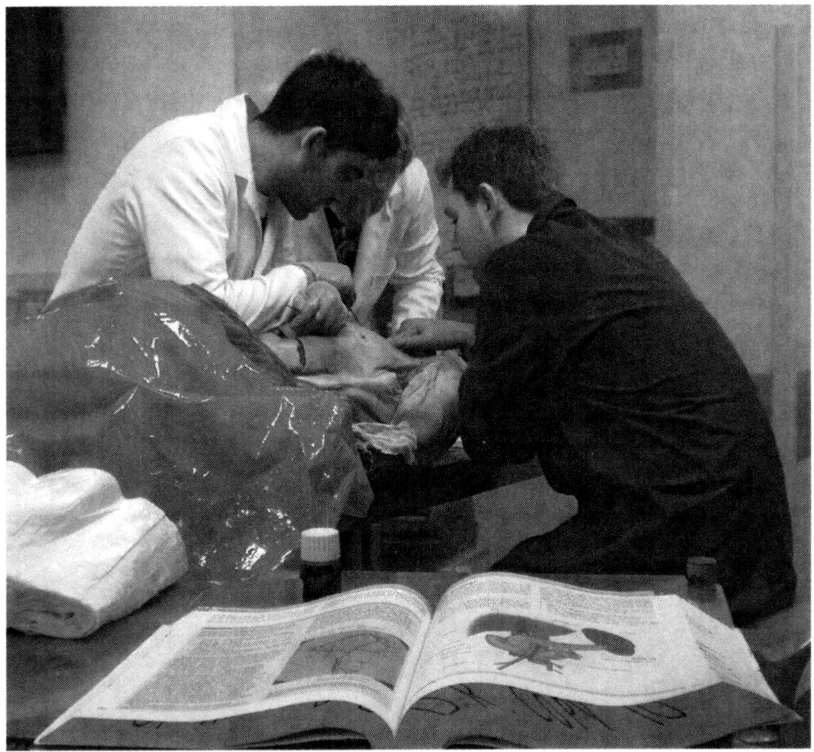

Figure 7.1 Newcastle University Anatomy Lab in 2012; photo by Rachael Allen

The act of inspecting and palpating a stranger's body, whether it is a live model or student peer, can cause embarrassment and unease. For some undergraduate students, placing their hands on another adult naked body is a highly emotional activity that can have an impact on their own sense of professionalism (McLachlan, 2004). If these emotions remain latent, the student is restricting the space for emotional maturity to develop through self-reflection, and without interaction, the student has no standard to realize the normalcy of these emotions.

Watching students close to dead human bodies makes for a profound observation: it is an acute scene. Students may feel challenged to find the most appropriate emotional level to deal maturely and professionally with sights unordinary to the public person. In his intensive study of a group of American students experiencing cadaveric dissection for the first time, Hafferty (1991) describes the cadaver as an "ambiguous man" and noted that levels of emotional discomfort rose with the uncovering or dissection of certain parts—the hand and arm, the head, the abdominal and the pelvic and perineal regions.

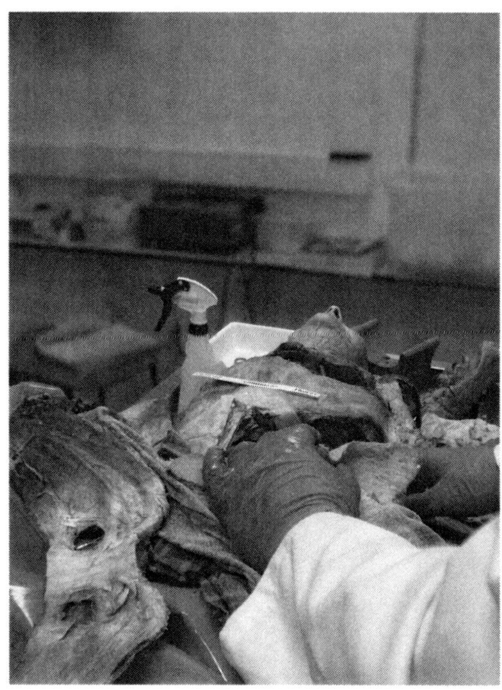

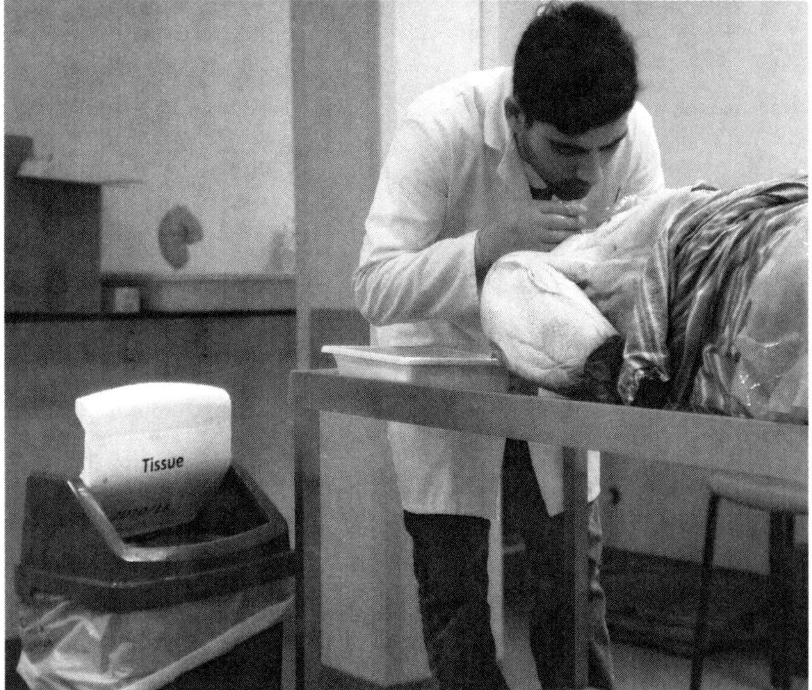

Figure 7.2 Newcastle University Anatomy Lab in 2012; photos by Rachael Allen

He concludes that this discomfort was caused by "the rather persistent re-emergence of the cadaver as a human referent" and suggests that students prepared to use this experience as a preventive from becoming overly cold and detached as doctors would have made an important step toward practicing as humane physicians (Hafferty, 1991). While this practice may provide a forum for students to develop a sensitive approach to death and dying, it may also help to reinforce the callous attitudes of others (Campbell, 2009, p. 110). Not every medical institute would agree that anatomic dissection or teaching from embalmed or plastinated specimens is a necessary component of medical training, and the debate on the value of such methods will likely continue among medical educators.

As an AIR I assume the unrestricted seat in the lab and surpass the field of view to observe body language, unspoken dialogue and the diminutive features of the environment that all bear significance to the experience of anatomy. Unqualified to make any judgments regarding the use of cadavers in undergraduate medicine, I can only respond to the experiences as an AIR and a human being. I feel moved when I overhear discreet comments shared among students while anatomy demonstrations are in progress: "I wonder what he died of?" and "How many children do you think she had?" and "Look at this scar!"

I consider the sensory experiences of the anatomy and clinical skills environments—the sight, touch, smell, taste and sounds—that are all responsible for stimulating the students' emotional and cognitive responses. More often than not, I see that these sensory stimuli go unrecognized or unacknowledged or are reduced to mere winces, grimace expressions or anxious blushing. It is these reactions that bear significance on students' anticipated response to future patients and their professional conduct within the clinical setting.

Specimen Life (Death) Drawing

As part of Project ANATOME, Specimen Life (Death) Drawing is a participatory workshop that engages medical students in the act of observing, drawing and tracing their visual, intellectual and emotional encounters in the anatomy lab. The session invites a group of first- and second-year medical students to draw still-life arrangements in the anatomy lab, including cadaver specimens and anatomy models. They spend 20 minutes on each arrangement before moving to the next station. After 80 minutes of drawing, they reconvene to discuss their experiences and share their drawings. The discussion encourages the students to talk about the thoughts and feelings initiated by the act of close inspection—a requisite for life drawing—and their general reflections on the workshop experience. Specimen Life (Death) Drawing offers the students an alternative encounter to that of the anatomy lab, one that I am privileged to witness through my observational work as AIR. The activity encourages them to look closely at the materiality of the specimens, the contrasting appearance (and nature) of cadaver and artificial models, and inspires conscious reflections on the presence of the donated specimen. The desired outcomes of the activity are to have the students' attention focused on the task of observation, rather than achieving drawing accuracy, and to offer an opportunity to discuss openly the concepts that capture their attention while they speak confidently about felt emotions.

Using drawing as a visual strategy for their observations bridges the gap between principal knowledge and sensory experiences of

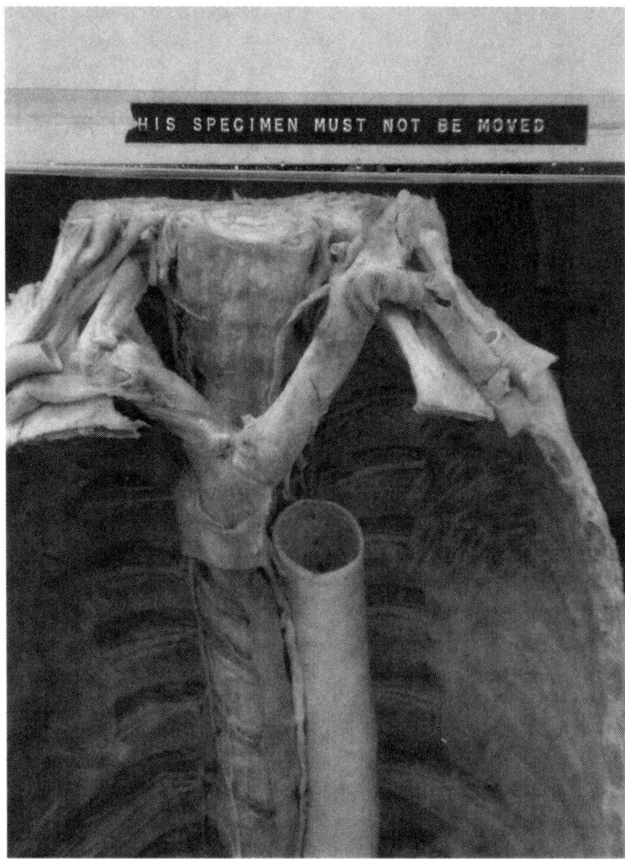

Figure 7.3 Newcastle University Anatomy Lab in 2012; photo by Rachael Allen

anatomy, giving rise to a more rounded, embodied, even humanized perception of the "dead" teaching the living.

Patient Study Module

Patient Study Module is a component of Project ANATOME, delivered in collaboration with Dr. Gabrielle Finn (anatomy lecturer) and Dr. Cathy Williamson (director of clinical learning). As part of the undergraduate medicine curriculum at Durham University, all first-year students take Patient Study and have the opportunity to observe the impact of chronic illness on an individual and his/her immediate family and/or caregivers in the community. The module provides a focus for the integration of learning in other strands of the curriculum in year two and further enhances team working, communication skills and ethical awareness.

Beginning in the 2013 academic year, first-year students and elected patients assigned to the Patient Study Module will be asked to volunteer as participants for the project sessions aimed at researching the role of art-making in generating visual interpretations of the patients' biological condition (as perceived by the student) and the personal experience of chronic illness (as conceived by the patient). Initially, I will attend two consecutive Patient Study meetings and passively observe interaction between student and patient. At the third meeting, I will introduce art-making activities for both participants, corresponding to the chronic illness specific to the study. Presented with a variety of materials and techniques including drawing, painting, collage, sculpture, writing and photography, the student will be instructed to create an artwork interpreting the patient's biological disease, and the patient to create an artwork expressing his/her personal experience of chronic illness. After the art-making session, time will be allocated for open discussion between student and patient. Each party will present the artwork to the other, exchange ideas, thoughts and feelings on their artistic outcomes and reflect on the overall experience. I will also invite both student and patient to participate in individual interviews to discuss their responses further. The outputs of these project sessions will also be considered for public exhibitions as part of Project ANATOME dissemination, on receiving consent from the creators, who remain the owners of the work. The module encourages patients to view their condition through a phenomenological lens, students through an anatomic lens, both responding to their visions artistically and ultimately sharing their artworks and perspectives. Similar to the Specimen Life (Death) Drawing workshop, the focus will be diverted away from the quality of consequent artworks and toward the process of listening, exchanging, understanding, questioning and developing visual languages.

The Patient Study Module incorporates the strand of medical humanities that advocates the use of arts and humanities to educate medicine. The activity invites student volunteers to transform their knowledge of gross anatomy and the principles of their patients' condition into a visual form using a creative process. Through this process, students can relate to the significance of thinking, seeing and "handling" their anatomic knowledge in a more creative way while remaining conscious of their patients' condition by referring back to their narrated symptoms and imagining their patients' internal bodies. To a degree, I am simulating a space for the students to revise anatomy principles in the presence of patients' illness experience.

The phenomenology of illness—that which privileges the first-person experience and challenges the medical world's objective account of disease (Carel, 2008, p. 8)—is the premise for the Patient Study Module, with the convergence of illness narrative and biological accounts. The student is being asked to render the disease of the patient's body—an object that can be weighed, measured and described—while accessing, acknowledging and appreciating it as a source of subjective feeling, sensations and perceptions. The activity introduces the student to illness phenomenology at a crucial point in their careers as doctors: the beginning. I invite students to read the work of Havi Carel, among others, who explores the phenomenology of illness in her book *Illness: The cry of the flesh* (2008) by weaving together the personal story of her own serious illness with insights and reflections drawn from her work as a philosopher. She writes,

> I quickly learned that when doctors ask "how are you?" they mean "how is your body?" ... they will not want to know how my life has changed because of my illness, how they could make it easier for me. (p. 39)

Illness narrative is a central theme that relates directly to another interest that inspires, and expands, Project ANATOME: the practice of narrative medicine. Emerging in the 1990s, this form of medicine is defined as being practiced with narrative competence and marked with an understanding of the complex narrative situations among doctors, patients, colleagues and the public. Dr. Rita Charon (2006), director of the program in narrative medicine at Columbia University, is a pioneer in the field and believes, "the growing scientific expertise of doctors needs to be aligned with the expertise to listen to patients, understand their ordeals of illness, honor the meanings of their narrated account, and to be moved by such so that they can act on the patients' behalf" (p. 3).

Picturing Diagnosis

Patient consultations require much more than physical examinations, lab results and diagnostic scans. Generalized medical knowledge must somehow be connected with the unique experience of the individual patient. The clues to diagnosis are often hidden in patients' habits, fears, beliefs and experiences, which can be accessible through the stories they narrate. Picturing Diagnosis calls upon the student as detective to investigate and diagnose anonymous conditions, with access to dramatic stories of real-life patients narrating debilitating symptoms, the challenges they face with medical treatment and the distress of bearing diagnostic errors.

The program was first delivered to a group of 25 medical students at Durham University in January 2013. I narrated 12 patient stories from various sources of modern literature—printed and web based—leaving the medical condition and terms of treatment anonymous. Laid out in front of the students were images corresponding to the details of the stories and patients' conditions, including clinical images (X-ray, MRI, ultrasound), anatomic images (diagrams, illustrations), medical equipment, patient appearance and a few red herrings, as well as anatomic models and clinical instruments. The students were required to listen to the patient stories, use their imaginations to associate the visual material with the details of the individuals' stories and eventually decipher the condition being narrated. In the true sense of narrative medicine, the activity draws students' attention to the act of listening and comprehending patient narrative to compose a pictorial map that will lead to a hypothetical diagnosis. The stories were also specially selected for their frank and unforgiving language, which helped to stimulate levels of empathy among the students and entertained the requisites of humane medical practice.

At the end of the session, I encouraged the students to share their thoughts and feelings in response to the activity and the narrated stories. They were provided with a bibliography of referenced literature exploring patient stories and narrative medicine to follow up outside of their curricular studies. Inviting students to embody the role of the doctor by listening to patients' stories highlighted the importance of grasping an illuminated view of another's experience, ultimately preparing students to practice with "diagnostic accuracy and therapeutic direction" (Charon, 2006, p. 11).

Artworks and Exhibitions

Project ANATOME, AIR activity and broader research culminate in mixed-media artworks presented in exhibitions and at academic conferences and disseminated through periodical literature. Entering the public domain, the art brings forth notions of how we come to know, see and experience ourselves in the world—our internal minds, external bodies and existential existence—by illustrating the biological, psychological and social facets of our universal human condition.

Death and Dissection, May 2012, Glasgow, Scotland

This exhibition was part of a series called *Let be be finale of seem*, presenting artists' work about death and the way it structures life. Inspired by my time as AIR in the anatomy labs, *Death and dissection* exhibited monochromatic drawings and miniature models that contemplate moral issues associated with the practice of human dissection and preservation and offer a view into the anatomy lab through a sensual screen.

The drawings in *Death and dissection* have their roots in observational studies. I sourced the drawings from sketches and annotations in my notebooks and exploited scale, composition and tone to marry the visual, intellectual and emotional encounters in the labs. Embalmed cadavers, prosected specimens, artificial models, mobile skeletons, "pickled parts" in jars and the teaching literature serve as a stimulating and assorted environment where the procurement of anatomic knowledge surpasses any other purpose or activity.

> The unforgiving aroma of formaldehyde is present where the stench of human decay should be. Even though their bodies appear discoloured, bruised, wounded, often burnt, they are fixed in a sphere that regulates deterioration. Besides the odd whiff of mould and dog-eared lung, the bodies are incapable of rotting the way nature intended. (Allen, n.d.)

The exhibition was received well by local medical students and academics, humanities scholars and the viewing public. I believe that closely juxtaposing anatomy education and notions of death and decay allowed medical students to contextualize their experiences in the anatomy lab and encounters with teaching specimens by acknowledging the important issues and ethics relating to death and dying. This acknowledgment helps to promote respect and gratitude toward people who donate their bodies to aid the medical studies.

Narratives of Medical Miniatures

I have exhibited medical miniature models widely throughout the past four years. Objects such as incubators and cots, hospital beds,

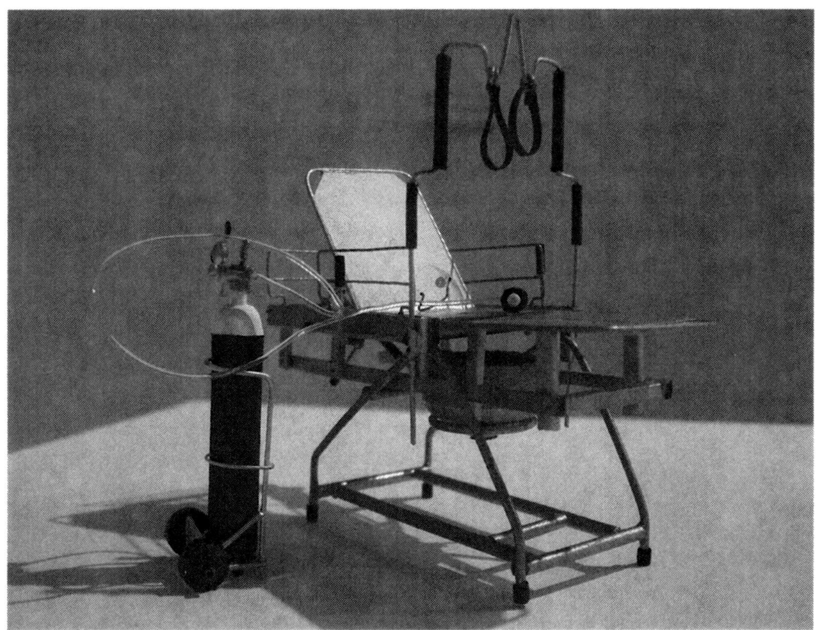

Figure 7.4 *Untitled (obstetric labour table and Entonox cylinder)* (2010–12), mixed media, 8.6 × 4.8 × 8 cm (dimensions variable); photo by Rachael Allen

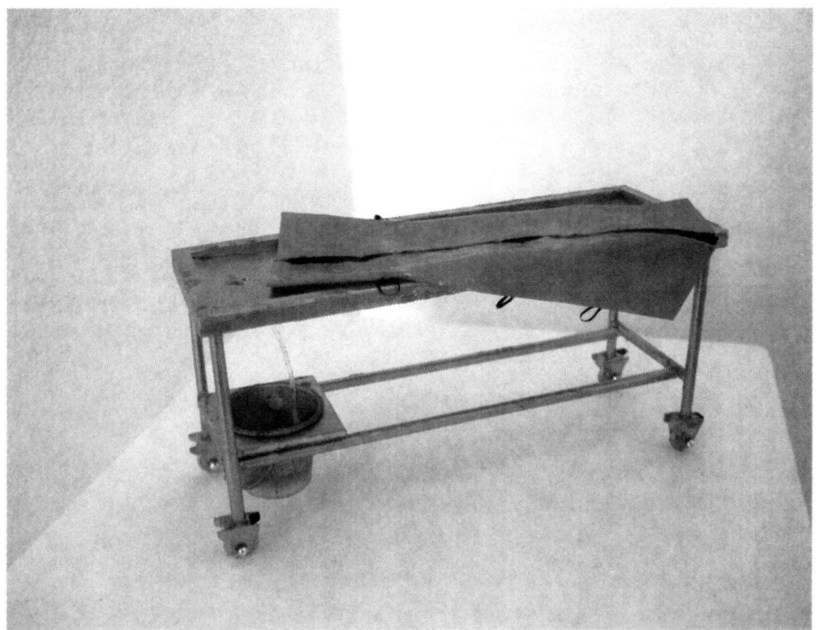

Figure 7.5 *Untitled (mortuary table)* (2009), mixed media, 5 × 4.2 × 11 cm, exhibited in *Death and dissection*; photo by Rachael Allen

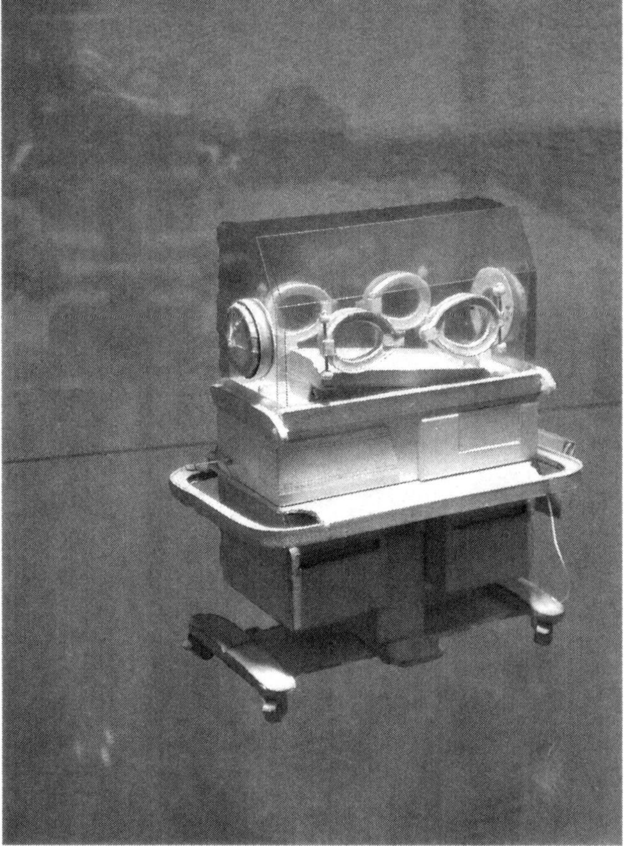

Figure 7.6 *Untitled (incubator)* (2008–12), mixed media, 6.5 × 4 × 9.2 cm, exhibited in *The waiting room*; photo by Rachael Allen

commodes, blood donor and chemotherapy chairs, and operating and labor tables are all receptacles for the patient body. Far from the immaculate condition of branded miniature furniture, these models wear the visible signs of medical use, bearing a doll's house pathos where the imaginary presence of the inflicted patient is implied by the absence of the miniature figurine. Each miniature medical model is a handheld metaphor for physicians' rigorous attention to the tools of their trade, treating a diagnosed condition in a practice that may be remote from the patient's own narrative.

If these miniature medical models had a voice, they would speak the language of pain, anguish, concern, frustration, conflict and dilemma that pervade the experience of medicine for patients, caregivers and often physicians. Medical students, academics and practitioners alike show great intrigue with these miniatures. For some,

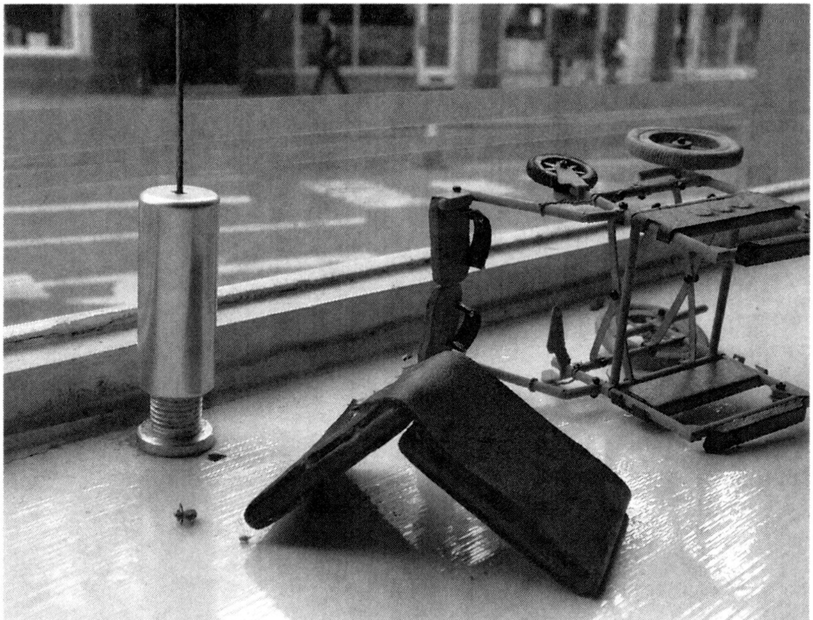

Figure 7.7 *Untitled (black wheelchair)* (2008–12), mixed media, 11 × 6.5 × 12 cm; photo by Rachael Allen

the objects evoke poignant memories from their history of specialties from obstetrics to pediatrics and from surgery to end-of-life treatment. In the same way literary work communicates the current affairs of medicine and the continuous reassessing of humane practices, the miniature artworks probe these issues by entertaining both our visual and intellectual perceptions and stimulate dynamic debates surrounding humane medicine from the terrains of both the (absent) patient and the practitioner.

The Waiting Room, September 2012, Newcastle Upon Tyne, UK

Inspiration for the artwork in this exhibition came from the wealth of research performed throughout Project ANATOME, from my time as AIR and from academic conferences. The examination of doctor–patient relationships—and indeed, the doctor and patient experiences of medicine—extends over decades and continues to stretch philosophical attention. In *The waiting room*, drawings and miniature models animate these philosophical notions, in the absence of professional debate and judgment, to serve visual slices of doctor–patient dynamics. The artworks address ethical concepts, questions and perspectives of medicine that have become part of contemporary culture today. Capturing the voice of patient and practitioner, the artworks

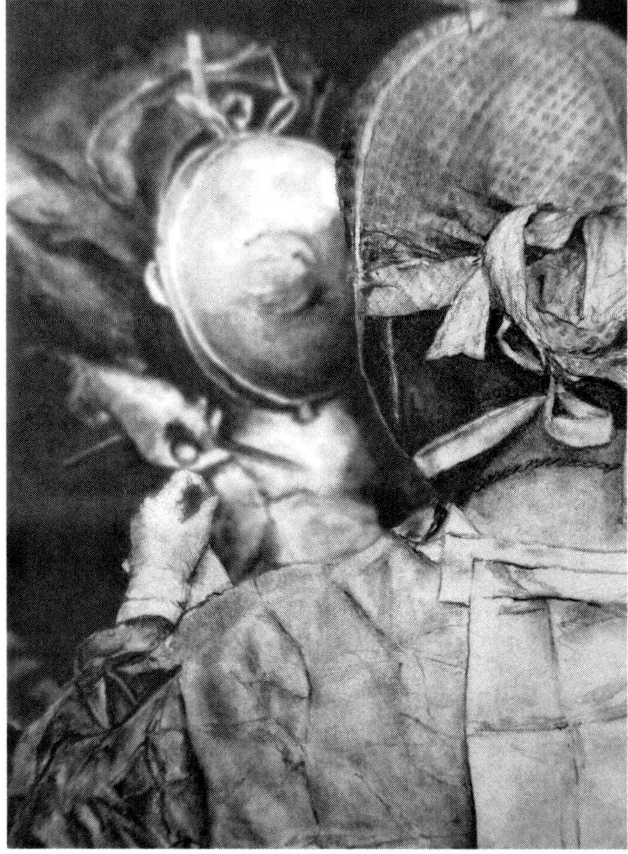

Figure 7.8 Detail from A3 drawing *Unclassified (BMJ 2007–2011)* (2012), extracts from British Medical Journal, pencil on paper, 3.5 × 2.4 cm, exhibited in *The waiting room*; photo by Rachael Allen

explore attitudes and perceptions of the doctor–patient relationship, exuding the concerns, frustrations, conflicts and dilemmas that pervade the experience of medicine.

The exhibition was received well by the public and the medical and humanities vocations alike. Once again, communicating with both medicine and the lay public is essential to creating a forum for the open exchange of thoughts, opinions and experiences, initiated by encountering the visual artworks. An artist talk accompanied the exhibition that furthered the discussions relating to the artwork. I delivered a supporting public lecture entitled "The art of illness," which was also selected for the multidisciplinary post-doctoral workshop "Body, corporeality and identity" at the Centre for Medical Humanities, Durham University. The paper presented the artwork of contemporary artists who represent illness in all its diverse variety: those who turn to creativity for tangible avenues of expression and who cope with the trauma of illness through art as therapy. The lecture invited open dialogues among those present—medical students, educators, artists and members of the public—regarding how one approaches artwork exhibiting illness and disease and to what extent these artworks extend beyond the nature of subjectivity and invite contemplation on what it feels to be human. Here, the value of visual artwork representing disease, illness and patients' experience of medicine was emphasized, and the opportunity to further discuss the role of art in medical humanities was offered.

I believe that in order for medical students to acquire a mastery of the body as a system of motion, but also emotion, they must access the sensual side of anatomy. To effectively treat (and mend) the body as a system that fails, but also feels, they must access their patients' stories. Artwork speaks to the mutual parties that constitute the grounds of medicine and clinical practice: people as life-long patients and medical students, educators and practitioners, all united in the exploration of the premises of humane medicine.

NOTE

My gratitude extends to all the medical academics and students at Durham, Newcastle and Northumbria universities who have offered their assistance and cooperation to Project ANATOME to date and have made it my privilege to assume the role as AIR. I am indebted to you all for your generous support and encouragement.

REFERENCES

Allen, R. (n.d.). *The anatomy lab.* Retrieved 2 January 2013 from http://www.rachaelallen.com/section623164_229108.html

Campbell, A. (2009). *The body in bioethics.* Abingdon: Routledge-Cavendish.

Carel, H. (2008). *Illness: The cry of the flesh.* Durham: Acumen.

Charon, R. (2006). *Narrative medicine: Honoring the stories of illness.* New York: Oxford University Press.

Coulehan, J.L., Williams, P.C., Landis, D., & Naser, C. (1995). The first patient: Reflections and stories about the anatomy cadaver. *Teaching and Learning in Medicine, 7*(1), 61–66. http://dx.doi.org/10.1080/10401339509539712

Hafferty, F.W. (1991). *Into the valley: Death and the socialization of medical students.* New Haven: Yale University Press.

Marks, S.C., Jr., Bertman, S.L., & Penney, J.C. (1997). Human anatomy: a foundation for education about death and dying in medicine. *Clinical Anatomy (New York, N.Y.), 10*(2), 118–122. http://dx.doi.org/10.1002/(SICI)1098-2353(1997)10:2<118::AID-CA8>3.0.CO;2-R Medline:9058019

McLachlan, J.C. (2004, Nov). New path for teaching anatomy: living anatomy and medical imaging vs. dissection. *Anatomical Record, 281B*(1), 4–5. http://dx.doi.org/10.1002/ar.b.20040 Medline:15558778

McLachlan, J.C. (2009, 4 August). *Flex and ply.* Retrieved 2 January 2013 from http://www.wellcome.ac.uk/News/2009/Features/WTX056102.htm

Rizzolo, L.J. (2002, Dec 15). Human dissection: an approach to interweaving the traditional and humanistic goals of medical education. *Anatomical Record, 269*(6), 242–248. http://dx.doi.org/10.1002/ar.10188 Medline:12467081

Stewart, S., & Charon, R. (2002, Mar 6). MSJAMA. Art, anatomy, learning, and living. *Journal of the American Medical Association, 287*(9), 1182. http://dx.doi.org/10.1001/jama.287.9.1182 Medline:11879121

8

Music as Medicine for Interdisciplinary Team Self-Care and Stress Management in Palliative Care

Amy Clements-Cortés

An occupation involving engagement with patients in palliative care can have serious mental, emotional and physical health effects on medical professionals. These professionals are busy with the day-to-day demands of their jobs and often fail to seek out resources to help them cope with the stress and loss in their environments. Music and music therapy hold the potential to assist medical professionals in multiple ways, including stress reduction and management, relaxation, dealing with feelings around clients' dying processes and dealing with bereavement and grief work. This chapter introduces the importance of self-care for medical professionals who may be experiencing stress, burnout and compassion fatigue, or grief and loss when working in palliative care. Music therapy is a treatment option to enhance coping mechanisms, reduce and manage environmental stressors and process grief and loss.

In this article I examine the foundations of music therapy and provide examples and clinical evidence of its efficacy in health care settings. I present environmental music and music-therapy techniques that may be used with medical professionals. I also provide narratives and examples of music-therapy sessions with health care professionals, with reference to lyric analysis, songwriting, improvisation and music for relaxation and stress reduction.

Stress and Palliative Care

Stress is defined as "any event in which environmental demands, internal demands, or both tax or exceed the adaptive resources of an individual, social system, or tissue system" (Monat & Lazarus, 1991, p. 3). Major sources of stress in the hospital environment include work overload, difficulties relating to other staff, problems nursing critically ill patients, anxiety and concern over patient treatment and patient condition (Dewe, 1989). The prevalence of stress in doctors, nurses, medical students and health care professionals is well documented, and stress can lead to job dissatisfaction and burnout (Deary, Blenkin, Agius, Endler, Zealley & Wood, 1996; McManus, Winder & Gordon, 2002; Bakker, Le Blanc & Schaufeli, 2005; O'Callaghan & Magill, 2009).

Self-care is extremely important for medical professionals working in palliative care. A variety of personal and environmental factors can lead to stress and burnout, and professionals whose personal and professional resources for handling work stress are limited are more susceptible to the effects of stress. Loss and grief are also major issues facing medical professionals and may contribute to burnout, emotional exhaustion, work stress and unhappiness.

Stressors unique to working in palliative care include dealing with patient deaths rather than cures, supporting entire family units (Hulbert & Morrison, 2006), involvement in decision making, the nature of the relationship between the nurse and the dying patient, workload and experiencing multiple losses (Vachon, 2000). In a study of palliative physicians' job stress and satisfaction, physicians reported that feeling overloaded was the greatest contributor to job stress, while job satisfaction came from having good relationships with patients, relatives and staff (Graham, Ramirez, Cull, Finlay, Hoy & Richards, 1996).

Burnout and Compassion Fatigue

Burnout is common among health care professionals (Embriaco, Papazian, Kentish-Barnes, Pochard & Azoulay, 2007) and is defined as "a syndrome of physical exhaustion including a negative self-concept, negative job attitude and loss of concern and feelings" (Keidel, 2002, p. 200). Compassion fatigue is similar to burnout but is associated with the stress that health care professionals experience when assisting a person who is suffering (Figley, 1995). With respect to hospice caregivers, Keidel (2002) outlined several factors that may lead to compassion fatigue or burnout, including personal characteristics of the care staff, patient and primary caregiver; societal influences; problems with the health care, institution, hospice or nursing systems; and stresses related to the patient's family.

Grief and Loss

Grief refers to the natural affective, physiologic and psychological reactions to losses (Brier, 2008). Granek, Tozer, Mazzotta, Ramjaun and Krzyzanowska's (2012) study of grief and experiences of loss among oncologists uncovered that the oncologists experienced sadness, crying and loss of sleep and harboured feelings of powerlessness, self-doubt, guilt, failure and responsibility for patients' deaths. Long-term care workers reported a wide variety of grief-related symptoms attributed to patient deaths, including sadness, crying, feeling unable to accept a patient's death and having trouble sleeping, and experienced negative effects on relationships with their own family members, co-workers and work (Rickerson, Somers, Allen, Lewis, Strumpf & Casarett, 2005).

The presence of environmental music and the use of music-therapy techniques may help health care professionals manage stress, resist burnout and compassion fatigue and cope with loss and grief.

Environmental Music for Medical Professionals in Palliative Care

Having music in the medical environment has proven effective in reducing stress and anxiety, improving communication and enhancing mood. For example, Cabrera and Lee (2000) found using music in a hospital setting to reduce noise pollution and aid in noise control helped reduce stress and anxiety for hospital employees. Furthermore, Ullmann, Fodor, Schwarzberg, Carmi, Ullmann and Ramon (2008) reported that when music was played in the background of a hospital, communication among staff was positively influenced; 63% of participants in the study listened to music regularly in the operating room and 61% of staff suggested that music should be played regularly. When Canga, Hahm, Lucido, Grossbard and Loewy (2012) used environmental music in a chemotherapy infusion suite and a waiting room, they found music helped address the needs of caregivers, medical staff, patients and families who might experience intense emotional stressors, and that environmental music was useful in addressing the effects of compassion fatigue in people caring for severely ill patients because the music reduced environmental noises and stressors and improved patients' and staff's moods.

Similarly, music listening has been shown to reduce stress in medical professionals. Allen and Blascovich (1994) found that when surgeons selected their preferred music to listen to during surgery, they demonstrated reduced autonomic reactivity and improved the speed and accuracy of performance of a stressful non-surgical laboratory task, compared to surgeons who listened to experimenter-chosen music or no music. Lai and Li (2011) established that when nurses listened to self-selected soothing music for 30 minutes, they reported lower levels of stress, cortisol, heart rate and mean arterial pressure, as opposed to nurses who were assigned to sitting in a chair and resting for 30 minutes. Attending music concerts also proved positive in reducing stress for dental students, and music listening was valuable in promoting physical relaxation and emotional self-regulation (Larsen, Larsen, Larsen, Im, Moursi & Nonken, 2012).

Music Therapy

The World Federation of Music Therapy (2011) states,

> Music therapy is the professional use of music and its elements as an intervention in medical, educational, and everyday environments with individuals, groups, families, or communities who seek to optimize their quality of life and improve their physical, social, communicative, emotional, intellectual, and spiritual health and wellbeing. Research, practice, education, and clinical training in music therapy are based on professional standards according to cultural, social, and political contexts. (¶2)

In medical settings, music therapy may be used with professionals to facilitate emotional expression, coping with grief and loss and improved quality of life while aiding overall health and stress management. There are numerous models of music therapy that music therapists follow in their practice or draw from to create a theoretical structure to guide their clinical work (Wheeler, 2012). The common thread among all models is that music is the primary tool to promote change in response to clinical goals and objectives.

Music therapy is a cost-effective, beneficial treatment option for medical professionals and health care organizations. Lavrova and Levin (2006) affirm music therapy is a psychological training method that helps reduce the level of burnout syndrome and increase the degree of personal effectiveness in participants. When studying the effects of music on self-reported stress levels and the immune system in the workplace, Brennan and Charnetski (2000) found music had a prominent and enduring reduction on participants' perceived level of stress.

Music-Therapy Techniques and Interventions

Music-therapy techniques may be categorized as receptive (listening), creative (composing), re-creative (performing) or improvisational (Bruscia, 1998). Receptive methods focus on the client listening passively to music and include interventions such as relaxation with music, visualization and imagery, music and collage, song-lyric discussion, vibroacoustic applications, music and movement techniques and other forms of aesthetic listening to music (Grocke & Wigram, 2007). Active methods include either structured activities or improvisational techniques. Improvisational techniques are achieved on a wide variety of instruments; specific techniques include mirroring, rhythmic grounding, containing, holding, frameworking and transitions (Wigram, 2004). Other active techniques of music therapy embrace song composition/songwriting, singing and playing instruments (Canadian Association for Music Therapy, 2012). Several of these techniques are beneficial in self-care as well as for treating stress, burnout, grief and loss.

Receptive Music Therapy

Receptive techniques in music therapy involve listening to music and/or reacting to live or recorded music (Bruscia, 1998). Music for relaxation is used in occupational settings to decrease the stress and anxiety associated with workplace pressures. Research suggests there is a cumulative effect from listening to relaxing music: Guzzetta (1989) reports that subjects' heart rates were lower after three music-therapy sessions, signaling the beneficial effects of music may be greater with repetitive use. In a study attempting to decrease anxiety levels in an occupational environment, Smith (2008) found that after a single session of music relaxation, participants' feelings of tension significantly decreased while feelings of relaxation and pleasantness significantly increased.

In the section that follows I outline three types of receptive music therapy: music relaxation, music and imagery and song-lyric discussion.

MUSIC RELAXATION

Music and relaxation sessions based on Grocke and Wigram's (2007) format begin with the music therapist assisting the client to become comfortable and adjusting client positioning and lighting while reducing noise and visual distractions. An induction follows to prepare the client for the music program. A variety of inductions may be used including structured/count-down, autogenic-type, colour, light and progressive muscle relaxation. Either live or recorded music follows the induction. Important elements in music for relaxation include a stable tempo, a stable volume or only gradual volume changes, reliable rhythm, timbre, pitch and harmony, a consistent texture, predictable harmonic modulation, appropriate cadences, predictable melodic lines, a repetition of material, structure and form, a gentle timbre and few accents (Wigram, Pederson & Bonde, 2002). Classical music is often chosen as it fulfills many of these criteria, but other types of music with different aesthetics (such as nature sounds or music from non-Western sources) may also be selected; sounds such as waves, birds and wind chimes or vocal toning, pan flutes, didgeridoos, African tribal drumbeats and sitars suggest the range of possibilities. The therapist then assists the client in returning to an alert state and engages the client in verbal processing and discussion of the experience.

MUSIC AND IMAGERY

Guided-imagery sessions begin similarly to relaxation sessions, with an induction followed by a music and imagery experience. Grocke and Wigram (2007) describe four different imagery methods: directed music imaging, which includes a script for the imagery; unguided music imaging, in which the client generates imagery in response to the music solely; group music and imagery, in which each group member generates his/her own response to music; and guided music imaging, in which the client engages in dialogue with the therapist to describe the imagery, and the therapist initiates questions and discussion. Following this discussion, the therapist assists the client in returning to an alert state and discussion often ensues to process the experience. The Bonny Method of Guided Imagery and Music (BMGIM) is a specific technique that requires advanced certification on the part of the music therapist (Lewis, 2002). McKinney, Antoni, Kumar, Tims and McCabe (1997) found that after taking guided-imagery and music sessions, participants demonstrated significant decreases between pre- and post-session measures for depression, fatigue and total mood disturbance, as well as significant decreases in cortisol level; they conclude that guided-imagery and music sessions have implications for chronically stressed people.

SONG-LYRIC DISCUSSION

Song and lyric discussion is another effective method of engaging medical professionals in discussing issues that cause stress at work.

Using the themes and emotions expressed in songs as a springboard, the therapist and participants are able to discuss issues indirectly and bring repressed or buried issues to the forefront. Addressing issues though music and the words of others is often less threatening than expressing them verbally outside of music's container (Clements-Cortés, 2004). With this intervention the music therapist may either choose songs before the session or may ask clients to choose songs that are meaningful to them for discussion. The focus of the song could be either matching where the client is that moment (focusing on stress, struggles, anxiety) or overcoming the trouble (recovery or stress release, for instance). Examples of songs used effectively in my clinical work in this area include "Candle in the Wind" by Elton John, "You Raise Me Up" by Josh Groban and "In My Life" by The Beatles.[1] After listening, the therapist and client can discuss the song's meaning or can pick specific lyrics and discuss their personal significance.

CASE: HEATHER, PERSONAL-SUPPORT WORKER

Heather is a personal-support worker who has worked in palliative care and oncology for more than 20 years. She participated in five individual music-therapy sessions I facilitated. This service was offered to health care professionals as a way to introduce music therapy in a new hospital program in Ontario. Through lyric analysis and discussion, Heather was encouraged to discuss her feelings of loss that accompanied patients' deaths and also the sense of loss and grief that is daily present on the unit. The song "I Will Remember You" by Sarah McLaughlin was particularly poignant for Heather, and we spent several sessions singing, discussing and improvising on the topics and feelings she expressed.[2] The last session was spent writing a tribute song for the patients she had worked with and lost to the melody of "Angel" by Sarah McLaughlin.[3] The following is an excerpt:

I'm in the arms of angels. They've flown away from here.
They are surely looking and watching over me.
We are born in this world where we live for a short time.
I will try to honour the lives of all that I see.

Creative Music Therapy

Creative music therapy offers a unique and therapeutic avenue for medical staff dealing with stress to compose or create music and write songs that address their issues and stressors to work through them.

CASE: MARY, HOSPICE PALLIATIVE CARE NURSE

Mary has been working as a palliative care nurse for more than 15 years. She was having increasing difficulty witnessing the deaths of the many patients she cared for. In individual music therapy, Mary was able to express her feelings, let out her emotions and talk about the stress and loss she was experiencing. The following is an excerpt from a song she wrote about the passing of several patients:

I am still alive and others around me die.
All that I can do some days is smile to ease their pain.
Take my hand and lift me up. I will help to guide you to your next land.
I hope that I have served you in the best way I can.

Mary had acknowledged how unhealthy it was to suffer in silence and not release her feelings. Music therapy enabled her to talk with the other nurses about her issues. This talk in turn opened an honest discussion in the group music-therapy sessions that were offered on a short-term basis to this interdisciplinary team. Together, through group songwriting and improvisation, they acknowledged patients who had passed and expressed feelings of anger, loss, confusion, gratitude and goodbye.

Re-Creative Music Therapy

Re-creative music therapy involves the client playing an already composed piece or playing various instruments in a structured way (as opposed to musical improvisation). Kuchinskas (2010) explains that stress starts in the brain and sets off a chain reaction of responses in every cell of the body, but playing music sets off an opposite chain reaction that switches the stress genes off.

Like health professionals, students in health and medicine experience burnout. They experience the stresses of student life combined with the emotional and psychological difficulties associated with working in a medical setting. In one study observing the effect of group drumming on first-year associate degree nursing students, Bittman, Snyder, Bruhn et al. (2004) found a 28.1% improvement in total mood disturbance and established that a typical student program of 105 students could expect to retain two additional students each year with the implementation of the music treatment. This improvement in retention rates would result in a projected annual savings of $29.1 million to nursing schools in the United States, a finding that shows that group drumming is not only psychologically helpful but also economically beneficial.

Singing can also be used as an intervention to reduce burnout, as singing has profound effects on emotion. Singing can induce states of relaxation, enhance physical health through improvements to breathing capacity, muscle tension, posture and the reduction of respiratory symptoms and contribute to social health through the management of self-identity and interpersonal relationships (Stacy, Brittain & Kerr, 2002).

CASE: JOAN, SPEECH-LANGUAGE PATHOLOGIST

Joan works as a speech-language pathologist with older adults in the rehabilitation and palliative care units of a large hospital. She has always enjoyed singing and joined a newly formed choir at the hospital, primarily because she wanted to keep up her music skills and perform. Belonging to this choir, which held weekly rehearsals, and preparing for a performance at an upcoming hospital event gave Joan the opportunity to socialize with other health care professionals, work as a team and reduce her stress. Singing each week contributed to her sense of well-being and improved her breathing, stress level and feelings of workplace satisfaction.

Improvisational Music Therapy

Improvisational music therapy is highly beneficial in exploring negative emotions and relieving stress. Hiller (2006) delineates between musical and clinical improvisation, explaining that musical improvisation is a process where individuals spontaneously create music while playing or singing to produce a musical product of aesthetic quality. Clinical improvisation is a process where the music therapist and client improvise together for purposes of therapeutic assessment, treatment and/or evaluation. In improvisation, the therapist and client choose a type of improvisation: free or based on a theme such as stress, exhaustion, release or relationships. After choosing appropriate instruments, the therapist and client engage in improvisation. A discussion often follows to highlight important events, thoughts or feelings that occurred during and after the improvisation. Lesiuk (2012) states that live instrumental improvisation can help provide psychological reversals, which is a stress-coping mechanism for individuals in high-stress occupations.

Transfer Effects from Patients to Medical Professionals

In many cases, music therapy targeted at patients results in benefits for the medical professionals treating the patients and can lead to reduced stress and work fatigue. O'Callaghan and Magill's (2009) study with oncology staff found that staff who experienced music-therapy treatment directed at patients described emotional and cognitive personal benefits and team benefits that in turn improved patient care. In experiencing the effects of music therapy for patients, staff experienced reduced stress and an improved work environment.

Conclusion

Health care professionals working in palliative care and medical settings face multiple stressors in their daily environments. This article has demonstrated how music and music therapy can be used in interdisciplinary team self-care to address the human needs of medical professionals by relieving stress, adding to intrapersonal understanding, helping to process grief and loss, and improving communication and teamwork among medical staff. Music therapy offers a unique and creative way to address issues specifically related to all aspects of self-care and not only is cost effective but also can provide long-lasting results.

NOTES

1 John, E., & Taupin, B. (1973). Candle in the wind. On *Goodbye Yellow Brick Road* [Vinyl Record]. London, UK: Trident Studios. Graham, B., & Lovland, R. (2002). You raise me up [Recorded by J. Groban]. On *Closer* [CD]. Reprise Records. (2003). Lennon, J., & McCartney, P. (1965). In my life [Recorded by the Beatles]. On *Rubber soul* [Vinyl Record]. UK: EMI Studios.

2 McLachlan, S., Egan, S., & Merenda, D. (1995). I will remember you [Recorded by S. McLachlan]. On *The brothers McMullen* [CD]. US: Brothers McMullen Productions.

3 McLachlan, S. (1997). Angel. On *Surfacing* [CD]. US: Arista.

REFERENCES

Allen, K., & Blascovich, J. (1994, Sep 21). Effects of music on cardiovascular reactivity among surgeons. *Journal of the American Medical Association, 272*(11), 882–884. http://dx.doi.org/10.1001/jama.1994.03520110062030 Medline:7811324

Bakker, A.B., Le Blanc, P.M., & Schaufeli, W.B. (2005, Aug). Burnout contagion among intensive care nurses. *Journal of Advanced Nursing, 51*(3), 276–287. http://dx.doi.org/10.1111/j.1365-2648.2005.03494.x Medline:16033595

Bittman, B.B., Snyder, C., Bruhn, K.T., et al. (2004). Recreational music-making: an integrative group intervention for reducing burnout and improving mood states in first year associate degree nursing students: insights and economic impact. *International Journal of Nursing Education Scholarship, 1*(1), article 12. Medline:16646877

Brennan, F.X., & Charnetski, C.J. (2000, Aug). Stress and immune system function in a newspaper's newsroom. *Psychological Reports, 87*(1), 218–222. http://dx.doi.org/10.2466/pr0.2000.87.1.218 Medline:11026415

Brier, N. (2008, Apr). Grief following miscarriage: a comprehensive review of the literature. *Journal of Women's Health, 17*(3), 451–464. http://dx.doi.org/10.1089/jwh.2007.0505 Medline:18345996

Bruscia, K. (1998). *Defining music therapy* (2nd ed.). Gilsum, NH: Barcelona Publishers.

Cabrera, I.N., & Lee, M.H. (2000, Apr). Reducing noise pollution in the hospital setting by establishing a department of sound: a survey of recent research on the effects of noise and music in health care. *Preventive Medicine, 30*(4), 339–345. http://dx.doi.org/10.1006/pmed.2000.0638 Medline:10731463

Canadian Association for Music Therapy (2012). Intervention techniques. Retrieved from http://www.musictherapy.ca/en/information/music-therapist.html

Canga, B., Hahm, C.L., Lucido, D., Grossbard, M.L., & Loewy, J.V. (2012). Environmental music therapy: A pilot study on the effects of music therapy in a chemotherapy infusion suite. *Music and Medicine, 4*(4), 221–230. http://dx.doi.org/10.1177/1943862112462037

Clements-Cortés, A. (2004, Jul–Aug). The use of music in facilitating emotional expression in the terminally ill. *American Journal of Hospice and Palliative Medicine, 21*(4), 255–260. http://dx.doi.org/10.1177/104990910402100406 Medline:15315187

Deary, I.J., Blenkin, H., Agius, R.M., Endler, N.S., Zealley, H., & Wood, R. (1996, Feb). Models of job-related stress and personal achievement among consultant doctors. *British Journal of Psychology, 87*(Pt 1), 3–29. http://dx.doi.org/10.1111/j.2044-8295.1996.tb02574.x Medline:8852018

Dewe, P.J. (1989, Apr). Stressor frequency, tension, tiredness and coping: some measurement issues and a comparison across nursing groups. *Journal of Advanced Nursing, 14*(4), 308–320. http://dx.doi.org/10.1111/j.1365-2648.1989.tb03418.x Medline:2661621

Embriaco, N., Papazian, L., Kentish-Barnes, N., Pochard, F., & Azoulay, E. (2007, Oct). Burnout syndrome among critical care healthcare workers. *Current Opinion in Critical Care, 13*(5), 482–488. http://dx.doi.org/10.1097/MCC.0b013e3282efd28a Medline:17762223

Figley, C. (1995). *Compassion fatigue: Coping with secondary traumatic stress disorder in those who treat the traumatized.* New York: Brunner/Mazel.

Graham, J., Ramirez, A.J., Cull, A., Finlay, I., Hoy, A., & Richards, M.A. (1996, Jul). Job stress and satisfaction among palliative physicians. *Palliative Medicine, 10*(3), 185–194. Medline:8817588

Granek, L., Tozer, R., Mazzotta, P., Ramjaun, A., & Krzyzanowska, M. (2012, Jun 25). Nature and impact of grief over patient loss on oncologists' personal and professional lives. *Archives of Internal Medicine, 172*(12), 964–966. http://dx.doi.org/10.1001/archinternmed.2012.1426 Medline:22732754

Grocke, D., & Wigram, T. (2007). *Receptive methods in music therapy: Techniques and clinical applications for music therapy clinicians, educators and students.* London: Jessica Kingsley Publishers.

Guzzetta, C.E. (1989, Nov). Effects of relaxation and music therapy on patients in a coronary care unit with presumptive acute myocardial infarction. *Heart & Lung, 18*(6), 609–616. Medline:2684920

Hiller, J. (2006). Use of and training in clinical improvisation among music therapists educated in the United States. Unpublished survey.

Hulbert, N.J., & Morrison, V.L. (2006, May). A preliminary study into stress in palliative care: optimism, self-efficacy and social support. *Psychology, Health and Medicine, 11*(2), 246–254. http://dx.doi.org/10.1080/13548500500266664 Medline:17129912

Keidel, G.C. (2002, May–Jun). Burnout and compassion fatigue among hospice caregivers. *American Journal of Hospice & Palliative Care, 19*(3), 200–205. http://dx.doi.org/10.1177/104990910201900312 Medline:12026044

Kuchinskas, S. (2010). How making music reduces stress. *WebMD the Magazine*, October 2010.

Lai, H.L., & Li, Y.M. (2011, Nov). The effect of music on biochemical markers and self-perceived stress among first-line nurses: a randomized controlled crossover trial. *Journal of Advanced Nursing, 67*(11), 2414–2424. http://dx.doi.org/10.1111/j.1365-2648.2011.05670.x Medline:21645041

Larsen, C.D., Larsen, M., Larsen, M.D., Im, C., Moursi, A.M., & Nonken, M. (2012). Impact of interdisciplinary concert series on stress and work–life balance in a dental college. *Music and Medicine, 4*(3), 177–187. http://dx.doi.org/10.1177/1943862112450188

Lavrova, K., & Levin, A. (2006). *Burnout syndrome: Prevention and management. Central and Eastern European Harm Reduction Network.* CEEHRN.

Lesiuk, T. (2012). *Reversal theory and music therapy: It helps being inconsistent! Psychological reversals and well-being in the workplace.* PDF retrieved from musictherapy.ca.

Lewis, K. (2002). The development of training in the Bonny Method of guided imagery (BMGIM) from 1975–2000. In K.E. Bruscia & D.E. Grocke (Eds.), *Guided imagery and music: The Bonny Method and beyond.* Gilsum, NH: Barcelona Publishers.

McKinney, C.H., Antoni, M.H., Kumar, M., Tims, F.C., & McCabe, P.M. (1997, Jul). Effects of guided imagery and music (GIM) therapy on mood and cortisol in healthy adults.

Health Psychology, 16(4), 390–400. http://dx.doi.org/10.1037/0278-6133.16.4.390 Medline:9237092

McManus, I.C., Winder, B.C., & Gordon, D. (2002, Jun 15). The causal links between stress and burnout in a longitudinal study of UK doctors. *Lancet, 359*(9323), 2089–2090. http://dx.doi.org/10.1016/S0140-6736(02)08915-8 Medline:12086767

Monat, S., & Lazarus, R. (1991). *Stress and coping: An anthology* (3rd ed.). New York: Columbia University Press.

O'Callaghan, C., & Magill, L. (2009, Jun). Effect of music therapy on oncologic staff bystanders: a substantive grounded theory. *Palliative & Supportive Care, 7*(2), 219–228. http://dx.doi.org/10.1017/S1478951509000285 Medline:19538805

Rickerson, E.M., Somers, C., Allen, C.M., Lewis, B., Strumpf, N., & Casarett, D.J. (2005, Sep). How well are we caring for caregivers? Prevalence of grief-related symptoms and need for bereavement support among long-term care staff. *Journal of Pain and Symptom Management, 30*(3), 227–233. http://dx.doi.org/10.1016/j.jpainsymman.2005.04.005 Medline:16183006

Smith, M. (2008). The effects of a single music relaxation session on state anxiety levels of adults in a workplace environment. *Australian Journal of Music Therapy, 19*, 45–66.

Stacy, R., Brittain, K., & Kerr, S. (2002). Singing for health: An exploration of the issues. *Health Education, 102*(4), 156–162. http://dx.doi.org/10.1108/09654280210434228

Ullmann, Y., Fodor, L., Schwarzberg, I., Carmi, N., Ullmann, A., & Ramon, Y. (2008, May). The sounds of music in the operating room. *Injury, 39*(5), 592–597. http://dx.doi.org/10.1016/j.injury.2006.06.021 Medline:16989832

Vachon, M.L. (2000). Burnout and symptoms of stress in staff working in palliative care. In H.M. Chochinov & W. Breitbart (Eds.), *Handbook of psychiatry in palliative medicine* (pp. 303–319). New York: Oxford University Press.

Wheeler, B. (2012). Five international models of music therapy practice. *Voices: A World Forum for Music Therapy, 12*(1).

Wigram, T. (2004). *Improvisation: Methods and techniques for music therapy clinicians, educators and students.* London: Jessica Kingsley Publishers.

Wigram, T., Pederson, I.N., & Bonde, L.O. (2002). *A comprehensive guide to music therapy: Theory, clinical practice, research and training.* London: Jessica Kingsley Publishers.

World Federation of Music Therapy (2011). *Announcing WFMT's NEW definition of music therapy.* Retrieved from http://wfmt.info/WFMT/President_presents..._files/President%20presents...5-2011.pdf

9

Expressive Arts and Practitioner Self-Care

Simply Being Human

Diane Kaufman, MD, Virginia S. Cowen,
Jodi Rabinowitz and Marilynn Schneider

So often in the medical setting there exists a disconnect between the patient as a person and the technological advances of medical practice. Health care practitioners may be encouraged implicitly or outright to put aside the inner self in favour of the "professional." Yet the inner self—and in particular the creative aspects of the self—does not disappear. Without adequate nurturance, practitioners are left feeling disconnected from themselves and the patients they aim to serve. Creative and expressive arts offer health care practitioners an avenue to form healing connections within themselves and their community.

Simply Being Human Expressive Arts Workshops for Healthcare Students and Providers, an Arnold P. Gold Foundation grant-funded research project at the University of Medicine and Dentistry of New Jersey (Newark), brings professional health care practitioners together and offers opportunities for participants to experience themselves as human "beings" instead of human "doings" as they connect with themselves, others and the natural world. Initial evaluation of the pilot program has provided information on how the workshops enrich participants' professional and personal lives. The goal for the program is to evaluate the impact creative and expressive arts can have in an urban academic health care community.

In our technologically advanced, rapid-speed medical practice, empathy, an important aspect of good clinical care, may be brushed aside in favour of efficiency. Setting aside emotions and inner creativity in favour of intellect can have a desensitizing effect on the health care practitioner (Bloniasz, 2011). When the creative and emotional aspects of the self are not nurtured, practitioners are left feeling disconnected from themselves, the patients they aim to serve and their colleagues in the health care community. Good health care relies on not only the ability of health care providers to connect with their patients but also on their ability to connect with each other (Garman, Corrigan & Morris, 2002).

In clinical education, empathy is a skill worthy of development. Recognizing and respecting a patient's feelings and experience are important components of patient-centred care (Shapiro, Morrison & Boker, 2004). In recent years, much attention has been given to the idea of including humanities in medical education, such as the exploration of literature, art and poetry related to clinical observational skills. Literature, in particular, offers the ability to investigate how something feels without actually having the experience (Moyle, Barnard & Turner, 1995). It offers the practitioner an opportunity to develop critical-thinking skills as well as empathy toward another's plight. Such skills are important when practitioners face the complexity and ambiguity often present in both art and the human experience (Gull, 2005).

Reflection is an important tool that can be used to promote and foster empathy. While the inclusion and intrusion of technology on health care practice has placed added demands on practitioners, the need for reflection still exists. As such, formal and informal opportunities for reflection must be part of clinical training (Hatem & Ferrara, 2001). This reflection includes reflecting on patient interactions.

Empathetic physicians may have healthier patients (Hojat et al., 2011). Although it is unclear why this relationship exists, it may be because patients are more willing to share information with a physician they perceive as empathetic, or because they are more likely to adhere to a prescribed treatment regimen. Creative methods in health care–provider education can help students understand the complexity of patient struggles and recognize the importance of expressing their own feelings (Milligan & Woodley, 2009; Shapiro et al., 2004).

There are many potential benefits to using creative and expressive art techniques to improve wellness in health care providers and students. Self-reflection through writing, storytelling, exploring poetry, making memory books and reading literature offers opportunities for therapeutic exploration and healthy self-expression (Bloniasz, 2011; McArdle & Byrt, 2001). Such self-expression can increase sensitivity and compassion during the activity itself and may also carry over into health care practice (Anderson & Schiedermayer, 2003). Increased attention to sensitivity and compassion can especially influence patient–provider communication, leading to better patient satisfaction and healthier environments. Health care providers and students who acquire new skills for creative expression are likely to use these skills as a personal and professional healing resource (Stuckey & Nobel, 2010).

Therapeutic relationships are reciprocal interactions between patients and health care providers. Even under the best of circumstances, the health care work environment can be stressful (Bloniasz, 2011). The psychosocial stress that affects health care workers has an impact on patients as well as on other providers and colleagues in the health care community. While efforts to promote worksite health generally focus on wellness for employees, a variety of interventions have been designed to attenuate psychosocial stress among health care workers. In particular, interventions often aim to provide a therapeutic outlet by focusing on workplace change, relaxation and creative activities (Marine, Ruotsalainen, Serra & Verbeek, 2006). The benefits of worksite group activities may improve not only individual well-being but also feelings of community and connection. Art therapy, for example, has the potential to build cohesive and therapeutic groups and to increase self-esteem when participants feel a sense of support and encouragement (Heenan, 2006). The creative arts also have the potential to forge connections among health care providers, caregivers and patients. When patients and caregivers have the opportunity to share their experience, health care providers' understanding and empathy increase (Colantonio et al., 2008; LoFaso, Breckman, Capello, Demopoulos & Adelman, 2010).

The experience of feeling connected to others is an important part of the healing process in therapy. Creative and expressive arts have a natural capacity to promote feelings of connection within groups of patients as well as within groups of health care providers. The sense of connection and the sharing of experiences and emotions can help providers feel more empathetic toward patients and colleagues. Writing poetry, for example, encourages participants to give voice to experiences and feelings; reading and performing poetry in a group furthers emotional exploration. It can also increase group cohesion, camaraderie and connection among group members (Kaufman & Goodman, 2010).

Several wellness programs have sought to include humanism in medical or nursing classes. Such programs have been advantageous for health care professionals who value skills such as empathy and compassion in addition to medical knowledge and technical acumen. In recognition of the many potential benefits of creative and expressive arts for health care providers and students, Simply Being Human was launched at the University of Medicine and Dentistry of New Jersey (UMDNJ). The goal of the program's expressive arts workshops is to create experiences that celebrate "simply being human" within a health care environment.

This program is not intended as therapy but rather as a method of creating support through the expressive arts within a community of health care providers. With the continued rise of technology in health care, there is no better time to commit to developing empathetic, compassionate, and creative health care practitioners. It is also a duty of the wider health care community to actively seek ways to diminish psychosocial stress and burnout in students and providers and to value nurturing in the caregiving community. These workshops and their subsequent evaluation not only provided participants an opportunity to explore together what it means to be a human who cares for other humans, but also provided objective measures to analyze the benefits of such an endeavour.

Designing a Creative Arts Series

The Society for Arts in Healthcare describes the creative arts in health care as a diverse, multidisciplinary field dedicated to transforming the health care experience by connecting people through the power of the arts at key moments in their lives—such as a serious hospitalization. The healing arts engage the patient's self through a variety of means, such as looking at pictures, drawing, sculpting, making jewelry, listening to music, making music, reading and writing poems, dancing or moving, to name just some of the many arts in medicine practices. Whether experienced passively or actively, the arts can serve as healthy distractions to the stress of illness and hospitalization. The arts can benefit health care students and providers in that the emotional and physical demands of working with the sick, which may lead to vicarious trauma and compassion fatigue, can be expressed, released and transformed through creative outlets (Society for the Arts in Healthcare, n.d.). The visual arts have been used to enhance observational and diagnostic skills, listening to jazz and appreciating improvisation skills has assisted in teambuilding and poetry has increased empathic connections with self and patients (Haidet, 2007).

This initiative at UMDNJ began through professional and personal connections with knowledgeable kindred spirits in and around a large, urban, academic health centre. Located in the inner city of Newark, the University of Medicine and Dentistry of New Jersey's University Hospital is the primary teaching hospital for New Jersey Medical School. The hospital is an essential health care safety net for the uninsured and under-insured. On the UMDNJ campus are many diverse and distinguished training, clinical, research and community outreach–oriented programs. These include but are not limited to the Healthcare Foundation Center for Humanism in Medicine, located within the Medical School; the School of Nursing's Center for Evidence-Based Practice; the School of Health-Related Professions; and the Institute for Complementary and Alternative Medicine.

There have been several initiatives to include creative and expressive arts in patient care and in activities to promote health care practitioner and student well-being. In 2008 the University Hospital received funding from the Van Ameringen Foundation to pilot supportive "healing" arts in medicine interventions for patients with head and brain injuries. Due to the severity of their injuries, these patients experience many physical and emotional challenges during their recovery. They may also be compromised in their ability to live independently compared with their pre-morbid way of life. The Planned Activity Less Medication (P.A.L.M.) room was developed as an "arts in medicine" approach to help enhance brain-injured patients' physical recovery and emotional well-being through scheduled activities such as music therapy, arts and crafts, movies, yoga, massage and other supervised projects, all taking place in a caring, personal and nurturing atmosphere (Theresa Rejrat, personal communication, December 31, 2012).

The seeds of Creative Arts Healthcare at UMDNJ were planted a year later in 2009. Dr. Diane Kaufman, Assistant Professor of Psychiatry and Pediatrics, a poet and an expressive-arts educational facilitator with expertise in the therapeutic uses of poetry, convened a meeting for health care providers across UMDNJ campuses who were interested in the role of arts in medicine. It was at this pivotal meeting that connections were made for arts in medicine practice to emerge more fully at UMDNJ. A creative synergy of shared vision, dedication and commitment was quickly established. The shared journey now had a name and a purpose: to establish Creative Arts Healthcare as a transformational change agent in health care practice by demonstrating the essential healing powers (both emotional and physical) the arts can have in fostering health in all its dimensions. To this end, Creative Arts Healthcare at UMDNJ was formed to educate students and staff on arts and healing, direct patient-care service, community outreach and research. The program was officially launched in January 2010 with the ultimate mission to "inspire and empower individuals to acknowledge, respect and transform the healing process through creativity" and the vision to "transform on a day-to-day basis the medical culture by recognizing and valuing creative self-expression as essential to health, healing, and humanistic care." A grant from the Society for Arts in Healthcare allowed Creative Arts Healthcare to seek guidance on program growth and development.

Activities include Grand Rounds, Poetry in Medicine Day, a poetry contest for health care students across all UMDNJ campuses, special events and performances. Events include musical recitals, writing workshops for nursing students and a presentation by a documentary filmmaker and an arts in residence program that serves hospitalized patients. Creative Arts Healthcare has received additional grants from the Institute for Poetic Medicine and the Arnold P. Gold Foundation. Faculty and staff who have contributed to Creative Arts Healthcare reflect an inter-professional group connected by their interest and belief in the healing power of the arts. The involvement of community artists in projects speaks to the connections possible with the community surrounding UMDNJ. Through these opportunities and connections, creative and expressive arts within the UMDNJ community and the University Hospital have blossomed.

The Workshops

The aim of the Simply Being Human workshops was to help health care students and providers to foster connections within themselves, patients, others and the natural world and to experience the vitality of these connections. Recruitment included e-mail announcements as well as flyers announcing the workshops posted throughout the hospital and medical school. Initially there was an enthusiastic response from the health care provider and student community. The workshops were to be scheduled one evening per month, and a spacious room at the Behavioral Health Sciences Building was identified as a meeting place. Invited guest artists facilitated workshops by assuming a leadership and mentoring role for the group members on their creative journey. Dr. Kaufman and Marilynn Schneider, both experienced in leading expressive arts groups, acted as support to these guest facilitators and also served as workshop facilitators for some of the groups.

The guest artists were recruited from the surrounding community in Newark, north-central New Jersey and New York City. Funding from the Arnold P. Gold Foundation supported the guest artists' workshop fees and the co-facilitators' fees. Faculty contributions, art supplies and space to hold the workshops were also donated.

During the workshops a variety of arts modalities were explored within the common theme of making connections. Each workshop blended group interaction with time for individual self-expression. The artwork belonged to each group member. The poems or prose written during the session would later, with member approval, be typed by the facilitator and shared with the other group members. Some examples of workshops are described below.

- **Connecting with the Self** was an initial welcoming invitation to take time for ourselves to "live, breathe and be" in the moment. There was an awakening of the five senses and a heightening of self-awareness. The workshop opened with guided meditation, relaxation and visualization and was followed by time to write, draw and share experiences. The group members felt supported to explore their inner landscape in a safe community.
- **Connecting with Self and Others** was a creative journey through movement, dance, poetry and drawing that explored the meaning and essence of the human experience. Participants began by modeling a simple movement that expressed "being human." These movements were choreographed into a dance that reflected each participant's expression of the human experience. Words were associated with the movements and shaped into a group poem. Participants then created drawings that reflected the movement, dance and poetry. Other workshops on this theme included poems embodied and "brought to life" through a sociodrama in which the group members both cast and directed their own writings with help and guidance from the guest artist, and a relaxing and almost meditative arts workshop activity in creating marbleized paper. Six-word memoirs were also added to the artwork. The focused attention of being in the moment and being one with the process was liberating.
- **Connecting with Patients** was a viewing of the PBS documentary *Healing Words: Poetry and Medicine.* This impactful film, which features the arts in medicine program at Shand's Hospital in Florida, interviews patients, family members, medical leadership, health care providers and also health care students. Using arts such as dance, music and poetry helped hospitalized

children and adults, as well as health care staff and students, not only to better express themselves but to experience a healing place within themselves; it also facilitated connections with others, increased understanding and helped create community. A group discussion of the film followed, as well as writing prose or poetry inspired by the film.

- **Connecting with Nature** explored the natural world through sounds and images evoked by music. After being given historical information on various musical compositions on natural themes, participants listened to the selections. While listening, they wrote down their thoughts and associations and drew images that were later used to form a simple poem. Participants were then introduced to a technique whereby they could follow the pulse of the music as they simultaneously re-read their poetry to deepen their experience of the music and words combined in an "entrained" or rhythmically synchronous manner.
- **Connecting with Nature and Living the Connections** was metaphorically expressed through the creation of three-dimensional collages. The arts activity sought to express each participant's life through images of sea, earth and sky. Participants learned to use a variety of principles and elements of art including shape, space, dimension and combination of materials. Each collage was a cosmos of nature imprinted with the participant's unique story. Participants used cut-out pictures and words and phrases to enhance their collages and made them three-dimensional by mounting them on foamcore boards. Members also learned from each other the multitude of ways that the materials could be used and that there was an endless supply of creative ideas. They experienced each other in new ways through telling their stories of nature and being alive artistically.
- **Living the Connections** used the poetry of Mary Oliver, William Stafford, Denise Levertov, Walt Whitman and Stanley Kunitz to explore the "thread of life." Packets of poems were prepared in advance and given to each group member. The poems were read aloud by the group members so the participants could hear the poems read in different voices. A discussion ensued, prompted by the words and images of the poems and the personal associations they triggered. As different poems were read, members commented on connections among poems and on how the poems spoke of life and its challenges. The group wrote a collaborative poem

> based on Mary Oliver's poem "The Journey," with each member adding a stanza to the poem. Their stanzas were first discussed and then the newly created group poem was read aloud, much to participants' delight and amazement. Copies of the group poem were later distributed to the group, further emphasizing "living the connections" both as an individual and as a member of a community. The experiences of meditation, visualization, breath work, stillness, listening and body work, as well as dance, music, visual arts and poetry, allowed for a heightened awareness of self. The inner being and its sixth sense of intuition can be nurtured through these processes, which give voice to a greater empathic understanding of self, patients and others. The desire to be more than just one's "fast moving and always doing" self is better realized and fulfilled by stepping back and allowing life to manifest through skills of quiet reflection and understanding. The health care students and providers practicing with these techniques were given the space to explore and experience the other without judgment, thereby creating a supportive environment.

Scheduling and commitment were challenging for some potential participants. During the first year, participants were asked to commit to attend the entire series of nine workshops. The biggest challenge for the pilot year was the small number of participants who were able to attend all nine workshops. Work, personal responsibilities, health issues and other challenges were intervening variables. Still, the workshops enabled a small number of participants to explore internal and external connections through creative activities. Having the same core group of participants in each workshop permitted a safe place to engage in creative exploration and to build on prior creative expressions and person-to-person connections made during the previous workshops.

Moving Forward

In many ways, the practice of medicine discourages creativity and individuality. Connections are purposeful and task oriented. Vital signs are taken, tests ordered, results reviewed. Forming meaningful connections is important for health care providers to remain empathetic and compassionate in their caregiving role. Theresa Rejrat, RN, MA, vice-president and chief nursing officer of Patient Care Services at the University Hospital, reflected on the importance of creative arts for health care providers, noting, providing care and service to the ill can be emotionally intense, inspiring and life changing. Health care providers often do not have the opportunity to talk about how this impacted them. The arts offer healthcare providers the opportunity to eloquently express in writings, poems or paintings, the tapestry of their own life experiences, a kaleidoscope of richly colored feelings, recognizing the beauty of their chosen career.

UMDNJ, a large urban academic health centre, was a fertile place to develop a creative and expressive arts program specifically for health care providers and students. The UMDNJ community has had several creative and expressive initiatives including, but not limited to, talent shows, exhibits of faculty, employee and student art in the hallways, and concerts performed by faculty members and guest artists. Despite the size of the campus, the variety of schools and the array of clinical services, creative arts were able to take root and grow. Building on these foundations, the Creative Arts Healthcare mission remains to "inspire and empower individuals to acknowledge, respect and transform the healing process through creativity." It aims to do this through education, direct clinical care, community outreach and research.

Simply Being Human, a humanism in medicine project, brought together health care providers and students to experience connections through creative and expressive arts. The art-making was the vehicle to foster connections with the self, create relationships with others, contemplate experiences of patients, experience nature and inspire harmonious living. By expanding the self's capacities through art, music, dance, movement and poetry, participants gained a greater awareness of creative strength and wholeness within themselves. Having participated in a creative act of their own making, they left the group with an expanded sense of self and an increased appreciation of creativity in their lives and the lives of others.

Because there was so much enthusiastic support for Simply Being Human from the group members in year one, funds remaining from the grant are being used to continue the project into a second year. The goal is to make creative and expressive arts for health care providers and students part of the fabric of the UMDNJ community. The journey of Simply Being Human Expressive Arts for Practitioners continues. For health care providers and students, this is a journey of health promoting human "doing" for patients, and also "doing" for self, integrated with an inner sense of human "being." The "doing and being" forms a tapestry of meaningful and compassionate connections we weave together even as we are being woven.

REFERENCES

Anderson, R., & Schiedermayer, D. (2003, Jun). The Art of Medicine through the Humanities: an overview of a one-month humanities elective for fourth year students. *Medical Education, 37*(6), 560–562. http://dx.doi.org/10.1046/j.1365-2923.2003.01538.x Medline:12787380

Bloniasz, E.R. (2011). Caring for the caretaker: a nursing process approach. *Creative Nursing, 17*(1), 12–15. http://dx.doi.org/10.1891/1078-4535.17.1.12 Medline:21462671

Colantonio, A., Kontos, P.C., Gilbert, J.E., Rossiter, K., Gray, J., & Keightley, M.L. (2008, Summer). After the crash: research-based theater for knowledge transfer. *Journal of Continuing Education in the Health Professions, 28*(3), 180–185. http://dx.doi.org/10.1002/chp.177 Medline:18712795

Garman, A.N., Corrigan, P.W., & Morris, S. (2002, Jul). Staff burnout and patient satisfaction: evidence of relationships at the care unit level. *Journal of Occupational Health Psychology, 7*(3), 235–241. http://dx.doi.org/10.1037/1076-8998.7.3.235 Medline:12148955

Gull, S.E. (2005). Embedding the humanities into medical education. *Medical Education*, 39(2), 235–236.

Haidet, P. (2007, Mar–Apr). Jazz and the 'art' of medicine: improvisation in the medical encounter. *Annals of Family Medicine, 5*(2), 164–169. http://dx.doi.org/10.1370/afm.624 Medline:17389542

Hatem, D., & Ferrara, E. (2001, Oct). Becoming a doctor: fostering humane caregivers through creative writing. *Patient Education and Counseling, 45*(1), 13–22. http://dx.doi.org/10.1016/S0738-3991(01)00135-5 Medline:11602364

Heenan, D. (2006). Art as therapy: An effective way of promoting positive mental health? *Disability & Society, 21*(2), 179–191. http://dx.doi.org/10.1080/09687590500498143

Hojat, M., Louis, D.Z., Markham, F.W., Wender, R., Rabinowitz, C., & Gonnella, J.S. (2011, Mar). Physicians' empathy and clinical outcomes for diabetic patients. *Academic Medicine, 86*(3), 359–364. http://dx.doi.org/10.1097/ACM.0b013e3182086fe1 Medline:21248604

Kaufman, D., & Goodman, K. (2010). Cracking up and back again: Transformation through music and poetry. In Z. Li & T.L. Long (Eds.), *The meaning management challenge: Making sense of health, illness, and disease* (pp. 117–129). Oxford, UK: Inter-Disciplinary Press.

LoFaso, V.M., Breckman, R., Capello, C.F., Demopoulos, B., & Adelman, R.D. (2010, Feb). Combining the creative arts and the house call to teach medical students about chronic illness care. *Journal of the American Geriatrics Society, 58*(2), 346–351. http://dx.doi.org/10.1111/j.1532-5415.2009.02686.x Medline:20374408

Marine, A., Ruotsalainen, J., Serra, C., & Verbeek, J. (2006). Preventing occupational stress in healthcare workers. *Cochrane Database of Systematic Reviews*, (4): CD002892. Medline:17054155

McArdle, S., & Byrt, R. (2001, Dec). Fiction, poetry and mental health: expressive and therapeutic uses of literature. *Journal of Psychiatric and Mental Health Nursing, 8*(6), 517–524. http://dx.doi.org/10.1046/j.1351-0126.2001.00428.x Medline:11842479

Milligan, E., & Woodley, E. (2009, Apr–Jun). Creative expressive encounters in health ethics education: teaching ethics as relational engagement. *Teaching and Learning in Medicine, 21*(2), 131–139. http://dx.doi.org/10.1080/10401330902791248 Medline:19330692

Moyle, W., Barnard, A., & Turner, C. (1995, May). The humanities and nursing: using popular literature as a means of understanding human experience. *Journal of Advanced Nursing, 21*(5), 960–964. http://dx.doi.org/10.1046/j.1365-2648.1995.21050960.x Medline:7602005

Shapiro, J., Morrison, E.H., & Boker, J.R. (2004, Mar). Teaching empathy to first year medical students: evaluation of an elective literature and medicine course. *Education for Health, 17*(1), 73–84. http://dx.doi.org/10.1080/13576280310001656196 Medline:15203476

Society for the Arts in Healthcare (n.d.). Society for Arts in Healthcare: Arts & Health. Retrieved January 9, 2013, from www.thesah.org/template/page.cfm?page_id=604

Stuckey, H.L., & Nobel, J. (2010, Feb). The connection between art, healing, and public health: a review of current literature. *American Journal of Public Health, 100*(2), 254–263. http://dx.doi.org/10.2105/AJPH.2008.156497 Medline:20019311

Lifelines

Medical Doodles

Drawing Toward Learning and Remembering

M. Michiko Maruyama

I was an artist and an industrial designer. To be honest, when I started medical school I was worried that I would lose my creativity. The opposite has occurred, however: through my medical training, I have become more creative.

At the end of each day, I sit and think about everything I have learned from morning to night and transform it into a Daily Doodle. For me, this is an act of reflection and a form of studying. The Daily Doodle becomes a condensed, pictorial version of my notes. It is the process of creating the Daily Doodle that consolidates my learning, and the actual doodle that is etched into my memory. After almost

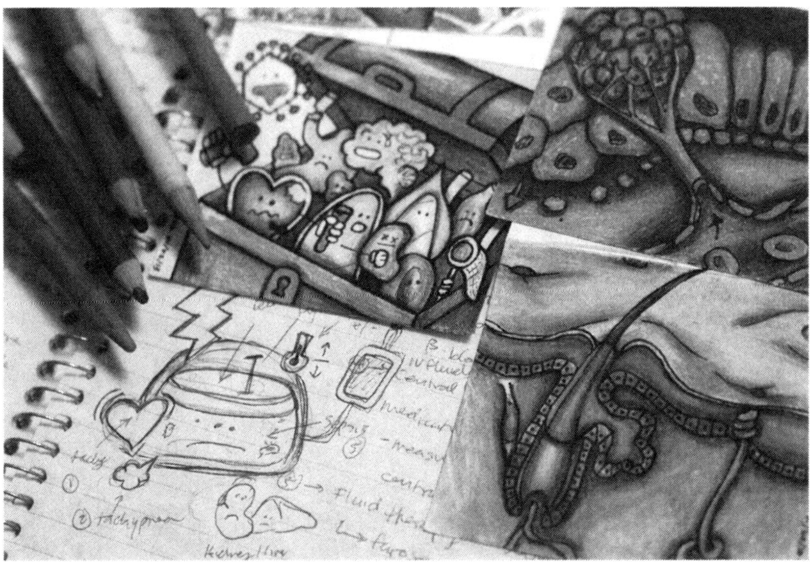

Figure L.1 A Daily Doodle by M. Michiko Maruyama

three years of medical school, my mind is filled with doodles that contain important information hidden within their lines and vibrant colours.

I started to post my Daily Doodles for my fellow classmates to see. After a set of finals, I received a message from one student saying that the student had recalled my doodles during the exam. Another student told me my doodles have become part of that student's learning process. Eventually I started to receive comments and messages from medical students around the world. A few weeks ago, a medical student in Pakistan e-mailed me to ask permission to use my doodles in a class presentation.

I am now in my clerkship year and even more pressed for time. Still, there is always time for a quick doodle, even if it is on the patient's chart to make note of an observation or to indicate the location of a laceration. Regardless of how busy I am, I make time for art and reflection because that's how I learn—and more important, that's how I relax and unwind.

NOTE

For more information about Daily Doodles, see Maruyama, M. (2012, Sep 4). "Medical doodles: 30 minutes well spent. Interview by Carol Ann Courneya." *Canadian Medical Association Journal, 184*(12), 1395–1396.

SECTION 3
NAVIGATING WITH NARRATIVE THROUGH LIFE EXPERIENCE

10

The Narrative Reflective Process

Giving Voice to Experiences of Illness

Jasna Krmpotić Schwind

It is a regular February day in southwestern Ontario … cold and windy with snow on the ground. I am going in for an annual physical exam. This year's exam is a little different in that my husband and I are preparing to start our family. I am giddy with excitement. Dr. Jones walks into the examination room. With his current practice at a local emergency room he is an expert diagnostician, the main reason I chose him to be our family doctor. He begins his systematic head-to-toe assessment. During these exams we usually chat about our common professional interest, emergency room care. This time, however, I am excitedly asking questions about the precautions I need to take with cat litter during pregnancy, when he suddenly stops and asks me to swallow. I do as he requests and then continue with my questions while he proceeds to palpate my neck. Dr. Jones interrupts me again and asks me to swallow. I swallow as his fingers gently press around my trachea. I know he is assessing my thyroid as he does every year. It is part of the routine check-up, I tell myself. However, I am mildly annoyed at the interruptions of my excitement when Dr. Jones, once again, asks me to swallow. I finally ask if there is a problem. He tells me he can feel a "little nodule" on the right side of my thyroid gland. The word "nodule" alarms me and my stream of questioning changes immediately to the newly presented data about my thyroid. "What do you think it is?" I ask. He responds cautiously that he is not too sure, but that it needs to be investigated. The weight of silence descends upon this medical encounter. The rest of the exam is a blur. My mood is subdued as I leave the office. In my head I am scanning all the possibilities. (Initial Diagnosis, Personal Journal Entry, Schwind, December 6, 2001)

ꕤ

I encountered this illness on two major levels: personal and professional. Jasna the person was scared of that illness whose name starts with the letter "c." She had heard stories of curtailed dreams and shortened lives by such sickness. Jasna the nurse-teacher knew the chances of having a malignant thyroid tumour and the options available to deal with it. Jasna was just in the process of teaching her students the peri-operative care of patients who undergo thyroid tumour surgery. She told them that the post-operative thyroid care was all a 'routine procedure' ... or was it? (Schwind, 2004)

Giving voice to patients' experience of illness gives us, the caregivers, in our diverse roles, a chance to glimpse the disease process from the other side. These illness stories create a doorway into the patient's experience of the disease, thus allowing the caregivers an opportunity to enhance the quality of meaningful person-centred care. In this chapter I share aspects of my illness trajectory to demonstrate how intentional and thoughtful reflection allowed me, as patient and caregiver, to make sense of the experience and, as a result, to alter my teaching–learning practices. I used narrative reflective process (NRP) (Schwind, 2008), a creative self-expression strategy that is informed by a narrative-inquiry approach to qualitative research (Clandinin & Connelly, 2000). What follows is an account of how my narrative inquiry into the illness experiences of nurse-teachers resulted in the creation of narrative reflective process. Components of this creative process—namely, illness stories and metaphors—are then illuminated. This section is followed by a how-to for the narrative reflective process. The chapter concludes with reflections on the value of narrative reflective process in health care education and practice.

Background

All life experiences, including those of illness, constitute who we are in our own evolutionary process. This claim is embedded in John Dewey's

(1963) assertion that "every experience enacted and undergone modifies the one who acts and undergoes, while this modification affects, whether we wish it or not, the quality of subsequent experiences" (p. 35). Connelly and Clandinin (1988, 1999, 2006) created the narrative-inquiry methodology by building on Dewey's philosophy of experience. They propose the following key assumptions: we access our experiences through telling stories of them; experiences consist of three dimensions: personal–social, landscape and time; and our personal and professional life experiences are intimately informative. These researchers suggest that when we deliberately construct a story of an experience, reflect upon it through the three narrative dimensions while considering called-for theories and bodies of knowledge (deconstruct) and then re-story the experience by including the newly gained meaning (reconstruct), the created narrative has the potential to inform our future ways of being, thinking and doing.

Narrative inquiry lent itself well in my research into the illness experiences of nurse-teachers (Schwind, 2004). I wanted to gain a deeper understanding of how our personal illness experiences affect our professional lives. At our first meeting, when I invited my co-participants to share their stories of illness, I quickly recognized what I was hearing was similar to the nursing reports on patient cases I was used to in clinical practice: professional facts, void of any emotion and personal impact. For our subsequent meetings, I decided to introduce creativity as a way to access our emotive responses to our respective illnesses. I found that eliciting patient stories through creative self-expression made visible the inner landscape of the ill person's hopes, fears and dreams, which were not yet accessible by words. This tacit knowing (Polanyi, 2009) revealed itself through metaphors, drawing and creative writing over the course of our meetings. Through this creative process we gave voice to our innermost selves, which were too premature for words, and so opened possibilities for new discoveries of meaning (Schwind, 2003).

Along with individual meaning-making of how the illness affected our personal lives, we also considered what our illness stories could teach us about our professional work. In my role as a researcher, using the narrative-inquiry data-analysis process detailed above, I read, re-read and deconstructed the stories and the creative self-expressions. Through this narrative reflection I came to understand the value and the place of patients' illness stories within therapeutic relationships. I also realized that we, as patients, feel cared for when our caregivers connect with our humanness. Consequently, when I returned to my role as a nurse-teacher, I envisioned a creative process that I could use in my teaching–learning situations to help my students—future caregivers—access their own humanness, so that they could then be available in more holistic ways to people in their care. I achieved this vision by formalizing my creative data collection with ill nurse-teachers into the narrative reflective process (Schwind, 2008).

Narrative Reflective Process

Narrative Reflective Process (NRP) consists of three key steps: story of experience, metaphor and creative writing. However, each step may be used independently, depending on the situation and the time availability. Thus, NRP can be adapted to any context where the intent is to increase self-awareness and personal knowing (Chinn & Kramer, 2008), as would be the case with caregivers and educators. It could also be used with patients when there is a need to make sense of their illness experience. For the purposes of this chapter I focus on the latter option.

Illness Stories

> *To seize the opportunities offered by illness,*
> *We must live illness actively;*
> *We must think about it and talk about it,*
> *And some, like me, must write about it. (Frank, 2002, p. 3)*

Illness stories are mechanisms through which we articulate ourselves and give meaning to our illness-disordered lives. Illness narratives, reconstructed stories of experience, are multi-dimensional, temporally contextualized within internal and external landscapes, and always exist in a relationship. By reconstructing our past in the present, we give our illness stories voice and open the space for dialogue. As such, "narrative offers a logic for explaining illness, provides metaphors for understanding the experience of illness and places illness and healing within human time" (Mattingly & Garro, 1994, p. 771). Each of our individual life stories, including those of a serious personal illness, "achieves its significance as part of a larger-scale experience or life story" (Sakalys, 2000, p. 1474) and accordingly contributes to a person's narrative unity (Connelly & Clandinin, 1999, 2006). It is the temporality of illness experience within its internal and external contexts of time, and physical and emotional space, that for me as a researcher, patient and nurse-teacher connects the illness story to the narrative inquiry.

Although illness stories have been documented as early as John Donne's 17th-century *Devotions*, their proliferation in book-length accounts occurred only in the latter part of the 20th century (Hawkins, 1999). This sudden increase in the focus on illness experience may be interrelated with the rapid technological advances and the biomedical model of health care that mushroomed in that same time period. As a result, objectified patients, their loved ones and many professionals—and more specifically health care professionals—turned to writing about the human experience of illness. We learn about these stories through different venues of expression: written accounts (Biro, 2010; Couser, 1997; Cousins, 1979; Fiore, 1990; Frank, 1997, 2002; Greenberg, 2009; Hawkins, 1999; Heshusius, 2009; Himes, 2002; Manguso, 2008; Winawer, 1998), dramatizations (Edson, 1999; Mitchell, Dupuis, Jonas-Simpson, Whyte, Carson & Gillis, 2011; Nisker, Martin, Bluhm & Daar, 2006; Pettle, 2000) and art and artistic exhibits (Cheng, 2010; Lapum, Church, Yau, David, & Ruttonsha, 2012; Mitchell & Halifax, 2005).

Health care researchers who study the experience of illness tend to scrutinize their patients' ordeals more so than their own. Rijke (1985), a medical doctor, researches the transformation and development of will in patients with cancer. As a physician and an anthropologist, Kleinman (1988) focuses on narratives of illness as experienced by those in his care and research work. Medical sociologists Davis and Horobin (1977) look at the illness experiences of their colleagues. Charon (2001, 2006), Greenhalgh and Hurwitz (1999) are medical researchers who investigate patients' illness stories with the intent to move the practice of medicine toward a more holistic approach to patient care.

No matter what form of expression they take, all illness narratives speak of an interrupted life, as if the threads of a tapestry are at the best snagged and at the worst ripped out. This sense of disorder permeates the patient's, and her/his family's, pre-illness world (Hawkins, 1999; Toombs, 1988). Constructing an illness narrative is an attempt to "discover, or create, a meaning that can bind it together again" (Hawkins, 1999, p. 3). This sense of disordering is poignantly illustrated in Winawer's (1998) and Edson's (1999) accounts.

Experiencing the illness of a loved one allows us a more poignant understanding of what it must be like for the sufferer. Winawer (1998), a gastrointestinal oncologist, observes after his wife becomes ill with stomach cancer "how utterly and completely people give up their individuality and control when they become patients" (p. 15). In his book *Healing lessons* (1998), Winawer confesses, "I experienced again that sense of disorientation from being on the other side [as] I was looking at cancer from a different perspective for the first time" (p. 34, p. 52). He had "faced cancer as a professional [but] never as a husband" (McLellan, 1998, p. 828).

This sense of role reversal brings forth for me an image of a mirror. In this image, I see how some health care providers put a mirror between themselves and their patients, thus obstructing a clear view between them. These caregivers seem to only see the reflection of their own needs and priorities, not those of their patients. I believe this scenario may also reflect Winawer, who, as a highly successful physician, was apparently treating disease out of context. That is to say that Winawer did not take into account his patients' human experience of cancer. However, this experience changed for him once the illness invaded his home and he experienced the role reversal from caregiver to care receiver. It was at this point that he was given the opportunity to look behind that mirror and to experience the illness from the other side. A line from Margaret Edson's play *Wit* (1999) aptly supports Winawer's sentiment. The patient named Vivian, a woman with end-stage ovarian cancer, remarks, "Once I did the teaching, now I am taught" (p. 37). Throughout the play, Edson communicates this notion of movement from one side, giving, to the other, receiving, by highlighting parallels between Vivian's professional life as a professor of 17th-century poetry and her personal life, being ill with cancer. In scene 10, after being tended to by a "young doctor," her former literature student, Vivian speaks to the audience:

> So. The young doctor, like the senior scholar, prefers research to humanity. At the same time the senior scholar, in her pathetic state as a simpering victim, wishes the young doctor would take more interest in personal contact.
>
> Now I suppose we shall see, through a series of flashbacks, how the senior scholar ruthlessly denied her simpering students the touch of human kindness she now seeks. (Edson, 1999, p. 58–59)

Winawer's work and Edson's work both resonate with my own experience of being ill. I have experienced the invisibility of being a patient and of being treated as a *disease* instead of a person who happens to be ill. When I was hospitalized, most of my caregivers did not introduce themselves either by name or by the role they played in my illness event. Their identification cards were certainly pinned to their uniforms, but most often turned around or tucked in the lab coat pocket, so their names were invisible. I captured that narrative thread in the following poem:

What's in a name?
Who are you?
What is your name?
Do you not care enough for yourself or for me?
Please see me!
I'm a human being too.
I am also someone's daughter.
I am also a healthcare provider like you.
Please let me see your humanness!
Please see mine! (Schwind, 2009)

The above accounts bring forth for me the awareness of our vulnerability as human beings and the way our need for human connection increases during serious illness. The social roles we seem to assume so easily can just as quickly slip away when the state of our health comes into question. At times like these our lives are turned upside down, and we try to tell or write stories about these disruptive events. We do so in the hope that some learning comes from our own suffering, so that fellow human beings following in our footsteps might have more meaningful experiences when they encounter turbulence on their own life paths. To that end many health care researchers, as I noted above, have dedicated their professional lives to exploring how patients' illness experiences might be made more meaningfully humane.

Kleinman (1988) strongly believes that medical relationships need to allow space for both "the science of treating disease and [...] the art of healing illness" (p. 223). Madjar (1997), a nurse-researcher, concurs with Kleinman's assertion that too often health care professionals tend to focus on the observable measurable aspects of patient care while neglecting the subjective, personal experience of the illness. She writes that "while disease affects the anatomical body, it is the person who experiences illness, who suffers, and whose embodiment is affected by bodily changes which go beyond the organic level" (Madjar, 1997, p. 57). Hearing how the patient experiences her medical predicament allows us to slip into her inner world: the "secret gardens of the self" (Williams, 1967, p. 288) "where the shape of suffering and the power of the healer's art lie revealed" (Daniel, 1986, p. 201).

To provide holistic patient care, we need to embrace both the personal patient experience of the illness and the technological treatment and support for it (Frank, 2010; Lapum, Fredericks, Beanlands, McCay, Schwind & Romaniuk, 2012). In Kleinman's (1988) sentiment, "each patient is a life story, and treatment means entering that peculiar life world" (p. 222). Therefore, restoring the patient's voice to the disordered biological function within the medical enterprise holds the greatest potential for holistic person-centred care. For health care providers, then, illness stories are a rich source of patient attitudes and cultural assumptions about illness, treatment and recovery and so can inform change that improves the lives of patients, families and caregivers (Charon, 2009; Hawkins, 1999).

Metaphors

Metaphor is a primary way for us to make sense of our experiences, especially overwhelming ones. Illness experiences are emotionally rich and are therefore more easily accessed and understood through the use of metaphor. When we struggle with traumatic events such as illness, metaphor helps us to access an intangible sensation or a painful memory by concretizing it in a manageable way, hence illuminating for us the meaning of that experience (Ritchie, 2010; Schwind, 2009; Shinebourne & Smith, 2010). Thus, in relation to the experience of a serious illness, the metaphor appears "to link thinking with feeling, [thereby bridging] the gap between the cognitive and affective domains" (Duit, 1991, p. 653). Metaphor helps us grasp the extraordinary in life by comparing it to the simpler—and, in the case of a serious illness, safer—alternative. It gives us a picture of our inner world of feelings and emotions and thereby a passageway into the experience that may be too nebulous to capture or too overwhelming to comprehend. Metaphor thus becomes another approach to explore emotions and emotional work for both patients and health care providers (Clandinin, Cave & Cave, 2011; Frank, 2011; Froggatt, 1998; Sharoff, 2009).

Sometimes we may have different or even apparently opposing metaphors for the same event. I believe this is due to the complexity of multifaceted experiences such as illness. Along with the explicit metaphors, we encounter the implicit metaphors that are embedded in each person's speech. Lakoff and Johnson (2003) propose that our conceptual system governs how we relate to our world within and without, and as such is central to how we experience and understand our reality.

To be useful, metaphor needs to be contextualized in bridging the meaning of the actual concept and the metaphorical one. Thus, the metaphor is inseparable from its experiential element, and it is "only by means of these experiential bases that the metaphor can serve the purpose of understanding" (Lakoff & Johnson, 2003, p. 20). It is important to stress, however, that the metaphor is not the situation. It is not the reality. Sontag (1990), who had been a patient herself, studied the existing language of illness metaphors in our society. In her writing she agrees that if we look at illness only through metaphor, we may jeopardize appropriate treatment. Although she acknowledges the role of metaphors in life, she fears that over time they may evolve socially to become a stigma that is more detrimental to the ill than the disease itself. Although I agree with this view, I also see the role of metaphor in a more positive light. Using the metaphor as a temporary tool that helps an individual span the gap between the actual situation of suffering and a less threatening one is beneficial as the ill person attempts to re-story him/herself in the aftermath of a serious illness. In this way illness metaphors serve a therapeutic purpose to patients at any stage of the illness process. Therefore, knowing when to release the metaphor becomes an art, unique to each individual undertaking this reflective process (Schwind, 2009, p. 20).

As caregivers we therefore need to inquire respectfully and thoughtfully and work with a patient's chosen metaphor. By exploring this with our patients, we look behind the mirror to learn not only how the illness event might appear from their side, but what questions and concerns they have and what clarifications they require. And, significantly, seeing the individual behind the disease places the person in the centre of our care, where together we are able to co-construct the therapeutic relationship. This way, the humanness of both the caregiver and the care receiver is honoured.

Here it might be useful to revisit the distinction between analogy and metaphor, as the two terms are often used interchangeably. Analogy has a partial similarity to the original situation or image and is "more logical and predictable, and in some ways linear, while metaphor is multidimensional, incongruous and capricious" (Schwind, 2009, p. 16). Although analogy is an excellent tool in teaching–learning situations, for the purposes of NRP, we are looking for a metaphor, an intuitively creative symbolic image. It is because metaphors are "simple in their brevity but complex in their unique meanings" that they hold the potential for "making sense of shared experiences" (Condon, 2012, p. 316).

Overview: The How-To of NRP

When narrative reflective process is used in its entirety, I begin by inviting the participants to write a story of an experience, such as an illness. It is important, however, to be sensitive about the readiness of the participants to engage in such an activity. For example, in my personal illness experience, I was not ready to engage in an in-depth reflection until several years had passed after the initial diagnosis. By writing about the experience we make its ontological dimension epistemologically visible and available for scrutiny. The personal story is then recounted to another person or, where possible, to a small group (ideally three). Each participant is given equal time to share her/his story uninterrupted while the other members actively listen. This sharing is often the first time the individual has had the opportunity to share the entire story with another human being.

The story is a gentle entry point, as that is how we articulate all of our experiences. The individual enters into the familiar space of putting into words what s/he is comfortable to express verbally. The story also creates a mental and emotional platform where images begin to form. From this space, I invite the participants to choose a metaphor, a symbolic image that best represents their illness. For example, in the study with ill nurse-teachers, Elizabeth chose a wolf to represent her life-long struggle with *Lupus erythematosus.* To further engage the creative process participants are asked to draw their metaphoric image and describe it to their group members, who are encouraged to ask thoughtful questions of clarification about the metaphoric image and its connection to the illness experience. For example, with the wolf metaphor one could ask: What feeds your wolf? How could your wolf be appeased? Through this supportive interchange, what was previously an inner feeling, and often confusing, is made socially visible, where "my experience" also serves to help others make meaning of theirs. If NRP is being carried out by an individual, then the multiple "I" of narrative inquiry (Clandinin & Connelly, 2000) allows for exploration and reflective dialogue from different perspectives. For example, when I wrote my illness story, I then stepped back into my researcher role and examined it as if it were another's story. After that, I looked at it from my roles of nurse-teacher, wife and daughter.

The final step of NRP is to engage in creative writing. I usually invite participants to have their metaphor write them a letter; if the metaphor could talk, what would it say? This request is often met with perplexed looks, but after this initial response the participants settle into writing the letter. Below is an excerpt of the letter my illness metaphor, "The Messenger Tumour," wrote to me.

Dear Mind-Body-Spirit, that is Jasna,

I know that your experience of being ill was not a pleasant one. It was like that for a reason. If everything went smoothly you would not have increased your insight into the patient's illness experience. ...

Now, you are finally coming into your own. Your authentic voice is emerging. The creative current is moving through your body once again. You are moving beyond me. I know you still fear the members of my family. That's OK. Just don't get too caught up in that. What will come, will come! Keep your faith strong. Keep your head and your body connected. Your neck is healthy now. [...]

Thank-you for giving me voice. Now I can leave you in peace. My job is done.

With blessings,
Your Messenger Tumour (Schwind, 2004)

Throughout the entire process, written stories, images, metaphors, drawings, conversations and letters are revisited and re-examined in light of each new insight. The temporality of narrative inquiry allows for this iterative process to move forward by critically looking back to explore our stories, make sense of them and so construct and reconstruct possible futures for ourselves (Lindsay, 2008). The reconstruction is always changing with each new experience (Dewey, 1963). Thus, we are always growing, evolving and creating. The new insights may be presented through reflective journals, poetry, poetic prose and any other form of creative self-expression. For example, after reading and re-reading my stories, my drawings and the metaphor letter, I encapsulated some of my key narrative threads in a poem. In the example below I write about the temporal evolution of my illness experience from my patient perspective:

Waiting ... Waiting ... Waiting

I wait in the waiting room
To see my family doctor.
Shock!
I have a nodule on my thyroid.
Test one.
I wait.
Inconclusive!
Test two.
I wait.
Inconclusive!
Test three.
I wait.
Inconclusive!
Surgery required!
I wait.

Conclusive!
The nodule is malignant.
I wait for radioactive iodine treatment.
I am isolated for three days.
I wait. I wait. I wait.
No caregiver checks in on me for the entire three days.
I wait for my voice to return.
I wait. I wait. I wait.
It takes months and years.
I wait. I wait. I wait. (Schwind, 2009)

This poem, along with my other writings, has become part of the performance narratives I use in my teaching–learning situations, as well as in workshops and conferences with my peers. Performance narratives add yet another dimension to the written text. The poetic performance narratives become the essence, a gestalt, like a metaphor of the entire experience, engaging emotionally and cognitively both me, the performer, and the audience.

Reflections

As human beings we are in a relationship with ourselves, our own life experiences and our cognitive, physical and spiritual world. We cannot not be in relationship. We are social beings, and we seem to look for this connection moreso when we are sick. How does this matter to health care education and practice? Relationships have the potential to be either healing or not. It is the quality of the relationship between the caregiver and the care receiver that matters. A caregiver who is also a patient is in a weakened state where s/he depends on the care of health care providers, her/his professional colleagues. If we as caregivers are disembodied ourselves and do not connect our minds with our bodies and our spirits, then we cannot provide opportunities for our patients to be whole human beings. If as caregivers we are uni-dimensional, then we cannot provide multi-dimensional beings the complete and proper care they deserve. The discordant relationship between the mind and the body affects the relationships between caregivers and patients. We can only be of service to our patients when we are in touch with our own humanness. The implication for health care education is, through role modeling and guidance, to help our students learn how to connect to their own humanness so that they too might more holistically engage with those in their care.

I question whether our health care curricula sufficiently address the whole person, not only in terms of the content but in the way we teach our students. I know that we have begun to teach holistic, person-centred care, but are we teaching it as holistic teachers, in a holistic way? I believe that learning is more effective when we are taught by example. What kind of an example have I been for my students? I think that to teach our students how to be holistic practitioners, we need to relate to them as such: mind–body–spirit. We may want to reflect on that notion and learn for ourselves the kind of role models we actually are for future practitioners.

Whatever I do in my life, I need to begin by looking at myself to learn who I am and what I bring with me into my personal and professional relationships. As an accountable nurse-teacher, I must acknowledge my own life's experiences, reflect upon them and understand how they shape my professional self (Schwind, Cameron, Franks, Graham & Robinson, 2012). By engaging my students in narrative reflective process, I open the possibility for them to do the same with their patients. Through this act, I believe that I move health care education and practice toward a knowing that exists beyond the theoretical and technical. I become caring. My relationships shift from the disease-oriented focus of I–It to the human experience of illness, the I–Thou (Buber, 1970/1996), where the sacred in each person is honoured and respected.

I reflect on how my own illness experience has moved from the individual to the social dimension, from the personal sphere to the professional one, and how this back-and-forth movement among dimensions of narrative inquiry moves my life forward, informing my teaching, through which I have the potential to affect the practice of future caregivers. In this way my own illness experience with cancer has found meaning in the greater social context of humanity, where other people's illness experiences might be made more meaningful and, as a result, their burdens a little lighter. Today, in my roles of nurse-teacher and narrative researcher, I guide my students and peers through the narrative reflective process of self-discovery and personal knowing (Schwind, 2008; Schwind et al., 2012). In this way these future caregivers more intentionally access their own humanness of care, making more transparent their unique narrative plotlines, ready to co-create mutually beneficial therapeutic relationships with their patients.

By knowing who we are and what we bring into our professional relationships, we become more whole ourselves. I hope that from reading my work, health care providers will be encouraged to think about their own life experiences—especially those of illness—and learn from them through reflection and reconstruction of those events; and further, that in this way they will encourage the same in their students and patients by providing space and guidance for that to happen. The student then no longer is a number and the patient is no longer "the gall bladder in room 453." We return to the original qualities of education and practice, those of competence, care and compassion for our fellow human beings. It is therefore less about teaching a new skill and more about shedding the conventions put upon us, the dominant paradigm of disconnection and separateness. It is about the restoration of humanness into our care, an innate dimension that is seeking to be given equal voice to that of science and technology. We need to keep in mind that "education is not just learning skills to make a living, it is learning to understand life itself" (Pettle's Thought for the Day, Tuesday, October 15, 2002).

REFERENCES

Biro, D. (2010). *The language of pain: Finding words, compassion, and relief.* New York: Norton.

Buber, M. (1996). I *and thou* (W. Kaufmann, Trans.). New York: Touchstone. [1970].

Charon, R. (2001, Jan 2). Narrative medicine: form, function, and ethics. *Annals of Internal Medicine, 134*(1), 83–87. http://dx.doi.org/10.7326/0003-4819-134-1-200101020-00024 Medline:11187429

Charon, R. (2006). *Narrative medicine: Honoring the stories of illness.* Oxford: Oxford University Press.

Charon, R. (2009). Narrative medicine as witness for the self-telling body. *Journal of Applied Communication Research, 37*(2), 118–131. http://dx.doi.org/10.1080/00909880902792248

Cheng, I.K.S. (2010). Transforming practice: Reflections on the use of art to develop professional knowledge and reflective practice. *Reflective Practice, 11*(4). 489–498.

Chinn, P.L., & Kramer, M.K. (2008). *Integrated theory and knowledge development in nursing.* St. Louis, MO: Mosby Elsevier. [1983].

Clandinin, D.J., & Connelly, F.M. (2000). *Narrative inquiry: Experience and story in qualitative research.* San Francisco: Jossey-Bass Publishers.

Clandinin, J., Cave, M.T., & Cave, A. (2011). Narrative reflective practice in medical education for residents: composing shifting identities. *Advances in Medical Education and Practice, 2,* 1–7. Medline:23745070

Condon, B.B. (2012, Oct). Metaphorically speaking. ... *Nursing Science Quarterly, 25*(4), 316–317. http://dx.doi.org/10.1177/0894318412457058 Medline:23087337

Connelly, F.M., & Clandinin, D.J. (1988). *Teachers as curriculum planners.* Toronto, ON: Teachers College Press.

Connelly, F.M. & Clandinin, D.J. (Eds.). (1999). *Shaping a professional identity: Stories of educational practice.* New York: Teachers College Press.

Connelly, F.M., & Clandinin, D.J. (2006). Narrative inquiry. In J.L. Green, G. Camilli, P.B. Elmore, A. Skukauskaite, & E. Grace (Eds.), *Handbook of complementary methods in education research* (pp. 477–487). Washington, DC: Lawrence Erlbaum Associates.

Couser, G.H. (1997). *Recovering bodies: Illness, disability, and life writing.* Madison, WI: The University of Wisconsin Press.

Cousins, N. (1979). *Anatomy of an illness as perceived by the patient.* New York: Bantam Books.

Daniel, S.L. (1986, Jun). The patient as text: a model of clinical hermeneutics. *Theoretical Medicine, 7*(2), 195–210. http://dx.doi.org/10.1007/BF00489230 Medline:3738845

Davis, A., & Horobin, G.G. (Eds.). (1977). *Medical encounters: The experience of illness and treatment.* London: Biddles Ltd.

Dewey, J. (1963). *Experience and education.* New York: Macmillan. [1938].

Duit, R. (1991). On the role of analogies and metaphors in learning science. *Science Education, 75*(6), 649–672. http://dx.doi.org/10.1002/sce.3730750606

Edson, M. (1999). *Wit.* New York: Faber and Faber, Inc.

Fiore, N.A. (1990). *The road back to health.* Berkley, CA: Celestial Arts.

Frank, A.W. (1997). *The wounded storyteller.* Chicago: University of Chicago Press. http://dx.doi.org/10.7208/chicago/9780226067360.001.0001

Frank, A.W. (2002). *At the will of the body: Reflections on illness.* New York: Houghton Mifflin Company. [1991].

Frank, A.W. (2010, Jan). Why doctors' stories matter. *Canadian Family Physician Medecin de Famille Canadien, 56*(1), 51–54, e39–e42. Medline:20090084

Frank, A.W. (2011). Metaphors of pain. *Literature and Medicine, 29*(1), 182–196. http://dx.doi.org/10.1353/lm.2011.0316

Froggatt, K. (1998, Aug). The place of metaphor and language in exploring nurses' emotional work. *Journal of Advanced Nursing, 28*(2), 332–338. http://dx.doi.org/10.1046/j.1365-2648.1998.00688.x Medline:9725730

Greenberg, L. (2009). *The body broken: A memoir.* New York: Random House.

Greenhalgh, T., & Hurwitz, B. (1999, Jan 2). Narrative based medicine: why study narrative? *British Medical Journal, 318*(7175), 48–50. http://dx.doi.org/10.1136/bmj.318.7175.48 Medline:9872892

Hawkins, A.H. (1999). *Reconstructing illness: Studies in pathography.* West Lafayette, IA: Purdue University Press.

Heshusius, L. (2009). *Inside chronic pain: An intimate and critical account.* Ithaca, NY: Cornell University Press.

Himes, M. (2002). *The sacred body: A therapist's journey.* Toronto, ON: Stoddart Publishing.

Kleinman, A. (1988). *The illness narratives.* New York: Basic Books, Inc.

Lakoff, G., & Johnson, M. (2003). *Metaphors we live by.* Chicago: The University of Chicago Press. [1980]. http://dx.doi.org/10.7208/chicago/9780226470993.001.0001

Lapum, J., Church, K., Yau, T., David, A.M., & Ruttonsha, P. (2012, Sep–Oct). Arts-informed research dissemination: patients' perioperative experiences of open-heart surgery. *Heart & Lung, 41*(5), e4–e14. http://dx.doi.org/10.1016/j.hrtlng.2012.04.012 Medline:22727038

Lapum, J., Fredericks, S., Beanlands, H., McCay, E., Schwind, J.K., & Romaniuk, D. (2012, Oct). A cyborg ontology in health care: traversing into the liminal space between technology and person-centred practice. *Nursing Philosophy, 13*(4), 276–288. http://dx.doi.org/10.1111/j.1466-769X.2012.00543.x Medline:22950731

Lindsay, G.M. (2008). Who you are as a person is who you are as a nurse: Construction of identity and knowledge. In J.K. Schwind & G.M. Lindsay (Eds.), *From experience to relationships: Reconstructing ourselves in education and healthcare* (pp. 19–36). Charlotte, NC: Information Age Publishing Inc.

Madjar, I. (1997). The body in health, illness and pain. In J. Lawler (Ed.), *The body in nursing* (pp. 53–74). South Melbourne, Australia: Churchill Livingstone.

Manguso, S. (2008). *The two kinds of decay: A memoir.* New York: Picador.

Mattingly, C., & Garro, L.C. (1994, Mar). Narrative representations of illness and healing. Introduction. *Social Science & Medicine, 38*(6), 771–774. http://dx.doi.org/10.1016/0277-9536(94)90149-X Medline:8184328

McLellan, M.F. (1998). The given moment. *Lancet, 352*(9130), 828. http://dx.doi.org/10.1016/S0140-6736(05)60733-7

Mitchell, G., Dupuis, S., Jonas-Simpson, C., Whyte, C., Carson, J., & Gillis, J. (2011). The experience of engaging with research-based drama: Evaluation and explication of synergy and transformation. *Qualitative Inquiry, 17*(4), 379–392. http://dx.doi.org/10.1177/1077800411401200

Mitchell, G.J., & Halifax, N.D. (2005, Apr). Feeling respected-not respected: the embedded artist in Parse method research. *Nursing Science Quarterly, 18*(2), 105–112. http://dx.doi.org/10.1177/0894318405274809 Medline:15802740

Nisker, J., Martin, D.K., Bluhm, R., & Daar, A.S. (2006, Oct). Theatre as a public engagement tool for health-policy development. *Health Policy (Amsterdam), 78*(2–3), 258–271. http://dx.doi.org/10.1016/j.healthpol.2005.10.009 Medline:16337306

Pettle, A. (2000). *Therac 25.* Toronto, ON: J. Gordon Shillingford Publishing.

Polanyi, M. (2009). *The tacit dimension.* Chicago: The University of Chicago Press. [1966].

Rijke, R.P. (1985, Jun). Cancer and the development of will. *Theoretical Medicine, 6*(2), 133–142. http://dx.doi.org/10.1007/BF00489658 Medline:4035607

Ritchie, L.D. (2010). "Everybody goes down": Metaphors, stories, and simulations in conversations. *Metaphor and Symbol, 25*(3), 123–143. http://dx.doi.org/10.1080/10926488.2010.489383

Sakalys, J.A. (2000, Jun). The political role of illness narratives. *Journal of Advanced Nursing, 31*(6), 1469–1475. http://dx.doi.org/10.1046/j.1365-2648.2000.01461.x Medline: 10849160

Schwind, J.K. (2003). Reflective process in the study of illness stories as experienced by three nurse-teachers. *Reflective Practice, 4*(1), 19–32. http://dx.doi.org/10.1080/1462394032000053521

Schwind, J.K. (2004). *When nurse-teachers become ill: A narrative inquiry into the personal illness experience of three nurse-teachers.* Unpublished doctoral dissertation. OISE/University of Toronto, Ontario, Canada.

Schwind, J.K. (2008). Accessing humanness: From experience to research, from classroom to praxis. In J.K. Schwind & G.M. Lindsay (Eds.), *From experience to relationships: Reconstructing ourselves in education and healthcare* (pp. 77–94). Charlotte, NC: Information Age Publishing Inc.

Schwind, J.K. (2009). Metaphor-reflection in my healthcare experience. *Aporia, 1*(1), 15–21. www.aporiajournal.com

Schwind, J.K., Cameron, D., Franks, J., Graham, C., & Robinson, T. (2012). Engaging in narrative reflective process to fine tune Self-as-Instrument of Care. *Reflective Practice, 13*(2), 223–235. http://dx.doi.org/10.1080/14623943.2011.626030

Sharoff, L. (2009, Oct). Expressiveness and creativeness: metaphorical images of nursing. *Nursing Science Quarterly, 22*(4), 312–317. http://dx.doi.org/10.1177/0894318409344760 Medline:19858507

Shinebourne, P., & Smith, J.A. (2010). The communicative power of metaphor: An analysis and interpretation of metaphors in accounts of the experience of addiction. *Psychology and Psychotherapy: Theory, Research and Practice, 83*(1), 59–73. http://dx.doi.org/10.1348/147608309X468077

Sontag, S. (1990). *Illness as metaphor and AIDS and its metaphors.* New York: Doubleday.

Toombs, S.K. (1988, Jun). Illness and the paradigm of lived body. *Theoretical Medicine, 9*(2), 201–226. http://dx.doi.org/10.1007/BF00489413 Medline:3413708

Williams, W.C. (1967). *The autobiography of William Carlos Williams.* New York: New Directions.

Winawer, S.J. (1998). *Healing lessons.* Boston: Little Brown.

11

Navigating Through Care

My Life Experiences with Medical Practitioners

John J. Guiney Yallop

The ambulance was late arriving.
It was your orders
or Dad's decision
or my screams
that put me in someone's car to St. John's
to the hospital
where I was given my nakedness
again
for the first time.

In this chapter, as a narrative inquirer and as a poetic inquirer, I navigate with narrative and ponder in poetry to explore my experiences with medical practitioners throughout my life: in my childhood, in my adolescence, in my young adult years and on into those ever-expanding middle years. I offer these stories and poems as my statement, my manifesto, about what I believe is important in the relationship between medical practitioner and patient. I also offer these stories and poems as gifts of gratitude, as hope for health care and, in some cases, as admonitions to attend for all who work in, make policy for and/or care about the practice of medicine.

I write in story and in poetry because story and poetry have been a part of my life from my early years and because it was to story and poetry that I turned as a researcher working in the field of education. Growing up in a small outport on the east coast of Newfoundland, I was surrounded by stories, both within my home and in the community. I also heard poetry, recited from memory; as an adolescent I wrote poetry to explore my emotions and to understand my experiences. When I decided to do a master of education degree, I used narrative inquiry, drawing on my own stories and the stories of two participants, to explore how gays experience school. Later, when I decided to continue my graduate research by doing a doctorate in educational studies, I used poetic inquiry to explore emotions, identities and communities; I examined my own emotions and identities as a gay person within and without communities. Writing narratively and poetically, usually autobiographically, has been my methodological approach to research. Story and poetry have also been healing journeys for me as I come to better understand my experiences and more fully embrace them … or vice versa.

I have lived with a myth since childhood, a myth from my own life, a myth about my first remembered near-death experience, a myth rendered poetically in the opening words of this chapter. It is a myth because I do not know how much of it is true, how much of it was invented in my memory as I have told and retold the story, and how much of it was invented in the memories of others as they also have told and retold the story about, or to, me. But something happened: I still have the scar on the lower right side of my abdomen where my appendix was removed. Did I have one hour to live, as I have recounted in the story so many times? Did my five-year-old body come near its end? In the one-hour drive from Admiral's Cove to St. John's, some of which was on a dirt road along Newfoundland's east coast, did my parents come close to losing their five-year-old seventh child after having lost their five-day-old first child? And was the doctor in the hospital who shouted at me as I begged him, through my tears, not to give me another needle, telling me to shut up, that he was not going to give me another needle, also the doctor who saved my life, who cut open my side to take out the sack of poison that would have exploded into my little body—and could have killed me? Why does the doctor who lived closer to us seem more gentle, at least in my memories, than the one in the hospital so far from my home? Is it because I did not see him, because I cannot even remember his name? I can remember the name of the doctor in the hospital, the likely surgeon—the one who screamed at me. Does screaming make one more memorable but less gently remembered?

Or do I recall more gently the doctor who lived not far from us because he did not hear my screams, did not come to our house (or did he?), did not have a chance to tell me to shut up (or would not have in front of my parents)? And the nurse who held me while I tried to pee, soon after my arrival at the hospital that night: why do I remember the relative safety of her embrace, a connection with another body among the sterile stainless-steel fixtures that defined that space?

Growing

In spaces of care
I live
with fear.

I have lived with fear all my life; to live with fear is not to live in it. Fear was present in that room in our outport Newfoundland home as I lay screaming for someone to stop the pain that stabbed at my side like a hot knife, siblings, parents, neighbours present, none knowing what to do and all seemingly powerless to end the agony. Fear was also present as I lay in that cot in the hospital in what we called town, St. John's, bandages covering the area above and to the right of my penis, marks from needles on my bum and arms—the latter where one needle remained to take fluid for food. I was living with fear and screaming my needs. Is that what I have been doing ever since, screaming my needs while living with fear? And are those responses I hear coming back at me now also screams, telling me to shut up, however well dressed they may be in political politeness and however well placed in positions of power? Hospitals are places where we come face to face with our naked vulnerability. We remember those experiences when we move in the world, where care can be a word emptied of meaning, while a scream, emptied of need, can be an action to shut us up and keep us in our place.

I have also known care as a living word, a word full of meaning. I have been living in care throughout my life. We use those words a lot: *in care*. We go into care. We put our children in care. We even address messages to someone in care of another. We all, it seems, live in care. The care I have lived in has come from family, friends, colleagues, communities as well as individual, and teams of, medical practitioners.

My living in care from medical practitioners began as I entered the world. I was born in a hospital, perhaps a first for my mother, who usually had her babies at home with the assistance of a midwife, perhaps her own mother because Mary Jane Harvey, my maternal grandmother, was a revered midwife in her community. I would return to that hospital just half a decade later to be taken into care again. This second visit, however, would also see me frightened by the man who had likely, as leader of the team of medical practitioners in the operating room, also saved my life. Hearing a scream come back at me, not out of any real need, just to put me in my place, to shut me up, left me feeling violated. It is an experience that has stayed with me, and one that I have used to measure the ethical behaviour of others, as well as my own behaviour.

I Lied About My Sight

Some people can say,
"I haven't told a lie in my life,"
although I think they might be lying then,
at least to the one who's talking,
but I can't say "I've never lied,"
not truthfully anyway:
My first lie in medicine was about my sight
when I wanted a new pair of glasses
in high school
because I was embarrassed about the free frames
I was wearing
since grade eight.
The optometrist caught me, however; those damn letter charts
don't lie.
"If you want a new pair of glasses, you just need to say so," he said,
and he probably meant it,
probably meant well, too,
but my just saying that would mean that mom would have to spend money,
money we didn't have.
When mom said, in a whisper, that I could get whatever pair I wanted,
I picked out a pair
and she paid for them,
or, I think she did;
I know that I've felt both grateful and guilty
ever since.

I dropped out of university more than two years into a bachelor of arts degree. Leaving was an emotional decision and experience. Perhaps in an effort to care for myself, I went to a dentist; I think it was the first time I had been in a dentist's chair. Unable to pay for the dental expenses that would accrue from the needed repairs, or for extractions of what was beyond repair, I arranged a plan-and-pay-as-you-go approach with the dentist. The dentist told me what needed to be done; I picked the most immediate needs, and we went forward from there. I felt no judgment of my poverty. Rather, I felt respected for the control I was taking both to understand my body's needs and to direct the care that would respond to those needs. Perhaps it is because a dentist's hands are in my mouth that I expect a careful attention to my voice, but in fact I expect the same careful attention whatever part of my body is being touched or entered.

When I moved to Ontario, after completing the degree I had walked away from, I injured my back while working with physically disabled men. After a few months of chiropractic care, I was heading back to work. My chiropractor advised me to reconsider; the advice was as much spiritual as it was medical. Perhaps that is what medicine needs more of, the spirituality of the shaman. "Listen to your body," that chiropractor said to me. "Was this an 'accident' or your body's response to a work situation that doesn't fit your body?" And then he added, "It's important to look back to learn, but we don't move forward by going back. In order to move forward, we need to also look forward and clear a path to our future by going forward." I resigned from my position as an attendant. Not long afterwards, I was hired as an educational assistant. Now, after my 30th year working in the field of education, that doctor's words continue to influence how I approach my life and work.

Silence = Death

It wasn't sex
that killed some of the men I've known
and loved.

Silence is an entry point for fear,
and fear keeps us silent,
and fearful silence doesn't use words,
and without words we have no voice,
and with no voice we cannot share
or negotiate
or agree (or disagree)
or be free,
and when we can't share
or negotiate
or agree (or disagree),
and when we are not free
we die
in silence.

My father died a good death, held in love and surrounded by family and friends. When I lived in Toronto in the 1980s, a good death was what many were trying to give those whose lives were coming to an end from AIDS. A population that was often characterized as the antithesis of family and community demonstrated to me what it meant to be a family and live in community. The vulnerable were cared for; they were touched—not touched as in moved by actions, but touched as in having the hands of another thoughtfully connect with their bodies. I recall being referred to a specialist for a medical condition that my doctor thought might be more clearly diagnosed if the specialist was aware that I was a gay man. "Patient is homosexual," my doctor wrote on the referral. In the specialist's office, I was very aware of touch—both that I was touched and how I was touched. Some years later, I was referred to another specialist. This time I wasn't touched, and the big oak desk between me and the specialist felt like a safety barrier—safety for the specialist. Another time, when I was in a doctor's office crying after experiencing discrimination and harassment, the doctor moved closer and held my hand. When I was moving to another city for employment reasons, I went in to let my doctor know about the move that would necessitate changing family doctors; I was hugged and thanked for the opportunity to have been part of my health journey. Another time, as I lay in an operating room, preparing and being prepared for a radical prostatectomy, a nurse asked me questions about my daughter and rubbed my arm and knee. She asked me if I was okay with this touching. I assured her that I was and that I believed touch was good.

Touch is likely a touchy subject in medicine, as it is in my field, and I understand and respect that bodies have boundaries as well as needs. "Don't touch the students," teachers are told. It's probably good advice, but good for whom? When we are in such need of touch, is it right to deny it? I learned to touch with a welcoming handshake, with a high five and with a smile that was also a smile from my eyes. Although eliminating or minimizing touch, beyond what is perceived to be the most necessary in medicine (or education), potentially, at best, minimizes risk of accusation of inappropriate or abusive behaviour, it also potentially minimizes the possible healing that is facilitated by touch. I have no easy solution, just a reminder of our common humanity.

Loving Care

The agony rose off my body,
pulled
into your hands,
its grip loosened
by a healer's love.

We don't use that word often,
and when we do

we look over our shoulder
for accusation
as if love
was a sin
or a crime
or a sickness
to be punished
or pitied.

While touch can be touchy, any mention of love can be muzzled. I want to be loved by those who care for me. I want to be loved, not in that dishonest religious rant of "Love the sinner, hate the sin," which comes in other variations: "Love the criminal, hate the crime" and, more applicable to this writing, "Love the patient, hate the disease." None of that is love.

I want to be loved with a love that is true and is truthfully expressed. I want to be loved with a love that connects me to another and connects another to me. I want to be loved with a love that embraces and that, while holding me in care, also frees me to live with care.

For over a decade now, I have been using the word *love* more freely, more openly, in my own field. At the most basic level of credibility, if I am going to call on practitioners in another field to engage in loving practice, and to speak of it, then I must also be prepared to engage lovingly in my own practice and use the language that expresses best what I do. I recall over a decade ago using the word *love* during a meeting about teaching. "The word has other meanings," I was told. "Indeed it does, but that doesn't have to stop us from (re)claiming the meaning it has for us in our practice," was my response. Later I heard the word used but with no notable change in practice. What I seek is congruence between my language and my practice, speaking of loving teaching, of loving my students, while also acting in loving ways as an educator in my work with students. I said at that meeting, "If we aren't loving our students, what exactly is it we are doing, and how are we doing it?" I would pose the same question to those who work in the field that is the topic of this book: If you aren't loving your patients, what exactly is it you are doing, and how are you doing it?

As I noted above, I offer these stories and poems with multiple motivations. I expect they will be received in even more ways than they are offered. Our lives are filled with stories and poems. Our lives are stories and poems. By attending to the stories and poems in a life, that make up a life, we come to better understand the needs of the person who is living that life. I would suggest that we also come to better understand ourselves, our own needs and our own lives.

12

The Childhood Novel and the Art of the Interview in Pediatrics Practice

Catherine L. Mah, MD

Novels offer us two forms of the narrative of daily life, suggests E.M. Forster (1927): the *life in time* and the *life by values*. Physicians, too, are chroniclers of human experience, passages through sequences of events. A medical encounter and, on a larger scale, a medical practice can and should also reflect the meaning of such experiences as well. Charon (2000) describes the parallel historical development of novels and clinical reports: both aim to "inspect and embody an individual human being's life and death within mortal time, giving full account of misfortune and suffering and engendering responses of both sympathy and identification in the reader" (p. 63). In this chapter I consider how the novel can be used as a foundation for narrative examination, through which physicians can learn to read and interpret the stories that are human experiences.

I will make two qualifications at the outset with regard to the conceptualization of creative arts in humane medicine. First, this chapter contemplates reflexive reading as a creative act, with reference to the ways in which narrative medicine takes the acts of reading and writing as intertwined and constitutive of a narrative practice. I will raise this point later with regard to the concept of intertextuality. Second, if the practice of medicine involves being active in prevention and treatment, then I wish to note that the discussion of humane medicine in this chapter highlights the example of one-on-one care, specifically the medical interview, but could also be relevant to a physician's relationship to populations, for example, in a community-medicine or public-health context. My observations, for example, stem from a decade in which I have transitioned from a primarily clinical office practice to a community-engaged public-health research practice.

Does reading novels make one a better clinician? I am not the first to ask this question (Little, 2003), nor likely will I be the last. What I propose here is that a close, reflexive reading of novels can prompt a physician to rethink how and why she observes and interprets events in the way she does. The idea is that the narrative of the novel, the narrative of the patient and the narrative of the physician may be considered in parallel as stories of human events, encounters, discourse, emotion, belief, motivation and action. Novels also take place in contexts: social, economic, cultural and political worlds. Examination of novels and other narrative forms allows physicians to better recognize stories, the way they are used in the everyday (Barthes, 1982), in lives and societies and in physicians' medical practices. In doing so, a physician can begin to develop what Charon (2001a; 2001b; 2006) has described as narrative competence, an "ability to acknowledge, absorb, interpret, and act upon the stories and plights of others" (2001a, p. 1897).

It has been argued that literature can be used to instruct, to evoke and to promote discussion, for example, among medical trainees about public health and social justice (Donohoe, 2009). I wish to go beyond this concept to suggest that the (creative) act of reading refines both observation and interpretation on the part of the physician. In other words, narrative competence can offer not only an entry point into a reflective and empathetic practice, but an evolving understanding that making sense of observations is a process that is *constitutive* of stories as well.

I focus on child health care. The pediatrician is unique in that in choosing to care for children, she chooses to celebrate life. To care for a child is to nurture the future potential of society through important transitions, on an individual and a population basis (Goldhagen, 2005). Well-child care, health promotion and illness prevention make up the majority of cases—disease and treatment, the minority. Of Forster's (1927) five "main facts" that comprise human life—birth, food, sleep, love and death—the pediatrician is an intimate friend of the first four and only an acquaintance of the last.

This chapter also considers the childhood novel, including novels for and about children. This is distinct from related inquiry on the role of literature directed toward child and youth audiences in medical practice (e.g., Bravender, Russell, Chung & Armstrong, 2010; Manworren & Woodring, 1998; Perrin & Starr, 2000). I offer illustrative examples from two Canadian novels, one classic and one contemporary. The former is the ever-popular *Anne of Green Gables* by Lucy Maud Montgomery (1908/1983), which centres on the character of Anne Shirley, an irrepressible orphan who manages to win over the community of Avonlea, Prince Edward Island, through both scrapes and successes. Emblematic of Canadian (rural) life and yet embraced by children of diverse cultures and environments, it is the first in a series of eight children's novels chronicling the life and times of Anne. While the works of L.M. Montgomery, including *Anne of Green Gables*, have been examined in great theoretical detail in the literature of children's literature (Siourbas, 2003), as far as I am aware a study of the novel has never been undertaken from the perspective of medical practice. It is also a novel in which I have personally been immersed since childhood with frequent re-readings.

As a contemporary counterpoint, I have selected Elizabeth Hay's (2000) debut novel, *A student of weather*. The work garnered several literary accolades when it was published. The book details 30 years in the life of Norma Joyce Hardy, a resilient "ugly duckling" who pursues the man she loves from 1930s Saskatchewan during the Great Depression, to Ontario and New York City through the Second World War. Both novels are "medically" bereft: disease events are few and far between. As I noted above, however, this lack of disease is not uncommon in the lives of most children, as pediatric caregivers know. What both novels do offer is insight into the processes of observation and interpretation. I will address these skills in particular within the context of the pediatric medical interview. In addition, both novels deal with the notion of expected behaviour, an assumption that frequently enters into childhood caregiving.

I begin with two passages that reflect first encounters:

> A child of about eleven, garbed in a very short, very tight, very ugly dress of yellowish gray wincey. She wore a faded brown sailor hat and beneath the hat, extending down her back, were two braids of very thick, decidedly red hair. Her face was small, white, and thin, also much freckled; her mouth was large and so were her eyes, that looked green in some lights and moods and gray in others. (Montgomery, 1908/1983, p. 11)

> She is eight years old. Afflicted by early puberty, penciled in by body hair ... Eight years old and still with all her baby teeth ... a tiny, out-of-proportion child whose forehead puts Elizabeth the First's to shame, whose earlobes could double as

pillows, whose baggy eyes could sleep an army ... Blue eyes ... smooth olive skin. (Hay, 2000, pp. 3–4)

A life in medicine daily includes such first encounters. As is often the case in the first pediatric medical interview, the children described above are introduced not at birth but at some significant point in their lives. For Anne, it is her first meeting with Matthew, her adoptive caregiver, who had expected to find a boy in Anne's place at the train station; for Norma Joyce, it is the moment immediately before her first encounter with the man she is to fall in love with, Maurice Dove. These first descriptions offer us tidy observations about the characters' basic appearances. Our characters are clearly rendered and yet, as readers, we are not satisfied. Should we be, as physicians?

Medical practitioners endeavour to glean, sort, order and effectively interpret "facts" from each patient encounter. In the case of documenting an illness event through a medical interview, we usually draw facts from focused observations—often derived from focused, or increasingly focusing, questions—and meticulous gathering of historical features. The description and contextualization of the event(s), compiled with an assessment of physical observations and other findings, point toward the diagnosis, or group of diagnoses, that is most likely. The awarding of a diagnosis leads to a decision about the appropriate management, and from then on, a re-evaluation of the patient's progress, a reference to existing knowledge about the condition, related conditions and best practices for management, to continue modifying diagnosis and treatment to the best fit. On a larger scale, the progress of many patients with similar events, diagnoses or management plans can be grouped into broader clinical experiences or research programs that will indicate the best management of future patients under similar conditions.

What if these "facts" are not so clear, however? What if the observations gathered in the initial encounter, albeit a thorough gathering, are but appearances that lead to assumptions about expected attributes, behaviour and outcomes? Observations without perspective, events as life in time, without value? What more can an "extraordinary observer" perceive?

From *Anne*:

an extraordinary observer might have seen that the chin was very pointed and pronounced; that the big eyes were full of spirit and vivacity; that the mouth was sweetlipped and expressive; that the forehead was broad and full; in short, our discerning extraordinary observer might have concluded that no commonplace soul inhabited the body of this stray woman-child of whom Matthew Cuthbert was so ludicrously afraid. (Montgomery, 1908/1983, p. 11)

From *Student*:

He had been taken aback by her ugliness, a word he modified to homeliness the next morning when she stood in his bedroom doorway and stared at him intently and at length; then at breakfast he thought her merely strange; and now, interesting ... It makes you think that boldness counts for more than beauty, and persistence counts for even more. (Hay, 2000, p. 26)

Here the practitioner is offered an opportunity. Beyond observation, the medical practitioner must make an interpretation. What these passages illustrate is that such interpretations depend not just on the basis of events gathered but also on the way the events are presented, and through that judgment alter the unfolding of the narrative itself. Each narrator reveals, through the eyes of our character observers, Matthew and Maurice, such information as may change our impression of the protagonists and our passage as readers through the story.

As Chatman (2000) has suggested about narrative point of view, we are guided by the "filter" of a character's consciousness as well as the "slant" of the narrator's voice. In a comparison of the texts, we see a differing level of involvement in the two observers, despite their formal positions as third-person narrators. The narrator in *Anne* stands back from the action, while the narrator in *Student* is omniscient, perceiving the inner workings of Maurice's mind. Both are able to provide extraordinary detail, albeit in different ways. For medical practitioners, the process of sorting through such layering in point of view in reading novels can provide practice in working simultaneously with inductive and deductive forms of reasoning.

I will come back to this point in a moment, with an examination of the pediatric interview process. First, let us examine *Anne* again. In the following passages, Anne speaks with Marilla, her stern but ultimately sympathetic adoptive caregiver and Matthew's sister:

"You're not eating anything," said Marilla sharply, eyeing her as if it were a serious shortcoming.

Anne sighed.

"I can't. I'm in the depths of despair. Can you eat when you are in the depths of despair?"

"I've never been in the depths of despair, so I can't say," responded Marilla.

"Weren't you? Well, did you ever try to imagine you were in the depths of despair?"

"No, I didn't."

> "Then I don't think you can understand what it's like. It's a very uncomfortable feeling indeed …" (Montgomery, 1908/1983, p. 26)

. . .

> "If you've finished your lessons, Anne, I want you to run over and ask Mrs. Barry if she'll lend me Diana's apron pattern."
>
> "Oh—it's—it's too dark," cried Anne.
>
> "Too dark? Why, it's only twilight."
>
> "… I can't go through the Haunted Wood, Marilla," cried Anne desperately. …
>
> "Fiddlesticks! There is no such thing as a haunted wood anywhere. Who has been telling you such stuff?"
>
> "Nobody," confessed Anne. "Diana and I just imagined the wood was haunted. All the places around here are so—so—commonplace …"
>
> Anne might plead and cry as she liked—and did for her terror was very real. Her imagination had run away with her and she held the spruce grove in mortal dread after nightfall. (Montgomery, 1908/1983, pp. 163–165)

To do justice to a child's narrative, a practitioner must use imagination. DasGupta (2006) has described how the imagination needed to deal with "complex, untidy, and confusing" (p. 457) storylines—in film, for example—is the same imagination physicians need to engage authentically and deeply with the stories of their patients, a process of co-authorship and not mere "elicitation" of stories. The imagination of the physician-reader goes beyond an empathy derived from close external consideration of perceptions and perceived experiences. Imagination is a form of active identification and creation of possibilities. For example, Wallace Hildick (1971), in early theory on criticism of children's literature, suggests that identification with a character is required to realize it fully. This interplay between self, narrative and creation of stories is central to medical practice. Put another way, imagination can be seen in both fiction and medical practice as a form of abductive reasoning, the creation of new hypotheses or narrative alternatives (Rapezzi, Ferrari & Branzi, 2005).

The pediatric narrative, in the setting of the interview, is an intricate one. By the age of six, many children are able to produce an easily understandable narrative of their own, and most pediatricians will come to rely on this information for a large part of their interview (Mendelsohn, Quinn & McNabb, 1999). Even before school age, children already have the desire to convey personal experience and to comment on the world around them, through narrative forms such as fledgling conversations, art and other creative media (Engel, 1995; 2005, p. 111).

In addition to the child's narrative, there is that of the caregiver(s), present or absent, and related family stories that impart meaning and norms (Wolraich, Wolraich, Dworkin, Drotar & Perrin, 2008, pp. 89–91). This range of texts and meanings means that all but a small proportion of pediatric medical interviews (e.g., with older adolescents or emancipated minors) are composed of, as a base, two—and often many more—narrative lines. This may not be unfamiliar to practitioners who engage with adult patients, but I emphasize that it is the *usual* circumstance in pediatrics. Pediatricians must also frequently deal with change. A child's age, developmental level and disease process will change, sometimes substantially, between one interview and the next, with the blending of and balance between child and caregiver narratives shifting steadily as the child grows and developmental capabilities are affected by health and illness states. In very rare circumstances, practitioners must even be alert to opposing narratives—or interpretations of such narratives—that can hinder attempts to engage with the child's personal narrative, for instance, in the controversial diagnosis of Munchausen syndrome by proxy (Baldwin, 2004).

Two concepts in narrative theory can assist here. The first is the idea of interpreting interwoven, interrelated and interdependent "texts," generally referred to under the umbrella of intertextuality, a term coined in poststructuralist literary theory of the 1960s and 1970s (Allen, 2000) that focuses on the configuration of meaning through the act and claiming of authority through reading, as opposed to writing (Fox, 1997). The second is the idea of narrative versions as described by Smith (1980), who argues that the production of versions of literary stories is not only about layering of interpretations on an "original" narrative but also about the multiple stories newly constructed in reference to the previous narrative, which can relate to it in multiple ways and meet the motivations and intended functions of the reteller.

If we apply these ideas to the pediatric medical interview, the presence of the immediately twinned child-and-caregiver (parent) narratives, which leads into processes of summarizing, inscribing and retelling by the practitioner, and the coalition of these texts as a whole will have an impact on the outcomes of the interview. These are manifest in each participant's interpretation of the illness and its experience, individual and collective decisions regarding therapy and medical record-keeping. What can be highlighted is that because the presence of multiple narratives is the usual starting point in pediatrics, unlike medical practice with adults, pediatric interviewing requires a particular sensitivity to the interplay among texts and the production of versions of accounts that are bound to occur in any single encounter. This sensitivity requires skills in detecting text and intertext, as well as narrative versions. As physicians in a strictly scientific medical role, we must sort through the details provided and retell the narratives as a unified whole—an interim "answer" to the medical "problem" at hand. As compassionate narrative practitioners, however, we also aim to preserve "original" perspectives alongside subtle nuances that make each of the individual narrative accounts unique. How can this be achieved?

First, let us consider the concepts of point of view and intertextuality in *Student*:

> He began to think the over-full lips less peculiar than sensuous, the over-wide forehead not outlandish but impressive, the licorice gums not so much weird but exotic. It can happen to anyone. You see the same plain landscape day after day, and then one day, perhaps it's the play of light or the time of year, you find it beautiful and other landscapes at fault. So it must be with fashion.
>
> ...
>
> Night after night Lucinda has poured one careful drop of lotion into her palm. Maurice watches her. Will she ever use more than one drop, he wonders. Will she ever have even one ounce of her sister's recklessness?
>
> Lucinda feels him watching and mistakes his curiosity for admiration, but it's only curiosity, and soon it isn't even that.
>
> ...
>
> Everyone's asleep except for the little gnome who slips out of bed and comes downstairs ... Finally, she draws out the ring. It's barely visible in the darkness, and quite cool. It spins loosely on her ring finger ... What she loved (besides his extravagance, which she loved most of all) was the way he smelled of the outside and inside, not just of air beyond the door but of train stations, bus depots, hotel rooms, restaurants.
>
> Besides that, the milky lower reaches of his neck and the soft flesh under his chin. Also his warm flexible voice. Also the way his tongue came down on a stamp.
>
> Norma Joyce Dove, she used to say to herself, nine times in a row. (Hay, 2000, pp. 89, 95–96)

Hay uses variations of the third-person narrator in these selections from part one of the novel. Three characters are involved—Norma Joyce, our protagonist, her sister, Lucinda, and Maurice, whom we have met previously, as well as a narrator or narrators' voice(s). Despite the suggestion that there is but a single narrator and several characters in the novel as a whole, we can see that in reality several narrative points of view—and narratives—come into play.

The first passage opens through the eyes of Maurice, seeing Norma Joyce, but Hay soon draws back and allows a narrator to comment on

Maurice himself: "it can happen to anyone." Following this, the narrative voice withdraws as far as a thoughtful reflection, an aside: "So it must be with fashion." Is this a reflection on the experience of the author herself? A text on fashion in the 1930s or the fashion world, volatile through history but only becoming "common" in the past century? The second passage reinstates Maurice as the primary observer with a new subject, Lucinda. A narrator's voice, however, arrives again, becoming intermingled with Maurice's own inner thoughts: "Will she ever use more than one drop?" "Will she ever have even one ounce of her sister's recklessness?" It is difficult to discern whether Maurice, the character, draws these conclusions or whether they are interposed by the insistent musings of the narrator(s). The final passage brings us back to our protagonist. This time, Norma Joyce is the observer, actor and thinker rather than the subject being observed. The narrator places Norma Joyce with Maurice's ring, found underneath the stove, where it had fallen. It "spins loosely on her ring finger," on which is described the features of Maurice Norma Joyce most loves. As in the previous passage, however, we witness a balance and mingling of character (Norma Joyce) and narrator consciousness: Norma Joyce has never been in a train station, or a bus depot, or a hotel room, or even a restaurant, and yet these are the "outside" smells she recognizes on Maurice. Where do these references arise? The final sentence suggests tentative admiration on the part of both Norma Joyce and the narrator, with Maurice's "tongue [coming] down on a stamp." Later in the novel, this brief suggestion of a stamp, of letters as narrative will return to haunt Norma Joyce.

As we can see, the depth of variance in perspective, relationship and retelling of perceived events is not uncommon in a novel. As readers, we can be trained to observe and interpret meanings embedded in such passages. Nor can the observation and interpretation of these meanings be separated from medical narrative. In a pediatric interview, for example, a child's narrative of an illness event could be considered alongside a parent's telling of the same events; a mother's memory and interpretation of a similar event occurring with a sibling, or in her own childhood; the family norms that shape the usual response to such events among kin or in the household; the teacher's interpretation and telling of the event to the mother at the school where, say, an infectious disease was contracted; the teacher's readiness or comfort to deal with illness in a child; and so on.

The other dimension at play is that of narrative versions. The mother's narrative about a child's illness experience can be viewed as not only her interpretation of what has occurred but a new version of the story that embeds her motivations in telling it in a particular way in the practitioner's presence. The same narrative can be rendered by the mother in a different version to a nurse, receptionist or medical student also engaged in the same encounter. The practitioner also develops a version while summarizing her interpretation of the illness at the end of the interview, and again in a medical record or transcription of the encounter. Like the novelist, in her creation of the story and its many voices, views and versions, the practitioner can use the possibilities of these multiple layers to cultivate a narrative awareness in her own work.

Developing a narrative sensibility is far from intuitive. Yet proficiency in narrative can optimize care of the patient and joy in the creative acts embedded in practice. Indeed, the novelist and the pediatrician—especially the pediatrician with narrative competence—are perhaps not far removed in their desire to cultivate and preserve stories of childhood for broader ends. The novelist begins with the child as he exists in life and goes on to create, in the child character, a microcosm of human progress in the larger world: in his infancy, our frailties; his illness, our struggles; his success, our resilience. The pediatric practitioner is witness to this progress in the everyday and has the opportunity to render narratives in tandem with that of his patient. On a larger scale, such narratives combine to produce cultural reference points about the innocence, vulnerability, freedom or promise of child experiences, sometimes referred to as archetypes of childhood (Jung, 1963; Byrnes, 1995). The archetypal child in medicine and literature is often a favourable reference, in that it embodies positive, "childlike" features—innocence, freedom, gentleness—as opposed to negative, "childish" ones. The archetypal child is also balanced with the notion of expectation, however, in the sense of possessing some proportion of "adult" perspective: wisdom, responsibility, adaptability, capacity, strength. In managing and, as I have argued in this chapter, actively creating such archetypes through stories, both the physician as reader and the writer of novels for and about children are active creators of what childhood represents.

REFERENCES

Allen, G. (2000). *Intertextuality*. New York: Routledge.

Baldwin, C. (2004). Narrative analysis and contested allegations of Munchausen syndrome by proxy. In B. Hurwitz, T. Greenhalgh, & V. Skultans (Eds.), *Narrative research in health and illness* (pp. 205–222). Oxford: BMA/Blackwell. http://dx.doi.org/10.1002/9780470755167.ch13

Barthes, R. (1982). Introduction to the structural analysis of narratives. In S. Sontag (Ed.), A *Barthes reader* (pp. 251–295). New York: Hill and Wang.

Bravender, T., Russell, A., Chung, R.J., & Armstrong, S.C. (2010, Mar). A "novel" intervention: A pilot study of children's literature and healthy lifestyles. *Pediatrics, 125*(3), e513–e517. http://dx.doi.org/10.1542/peds.2009-1666 Medline:20142279

Byrnes, A. (1995). *The child: An archetypal symbol in literature for children and adults.* New York: Peter Larry Publishing, Inc.

Charon, R. (2000, Jan 4). Medicine, the novel, and the passage of time. *Annals of Internal Medicine, 132*(1), 63–68. http://dx.doi.org/10.7326/0003-4819-132-1-200001040-00011 Medline:10627254

Charon, R. (2001a, Oct 17). The patient–physician relationship. Narrative medicine: a model for empathy, reflection, profession, and trust. *Journal of the American Medical Association, 286*(15), 1897–1902. http://dx.doi.org/10.1001/jama.286.15.1897 Medline:11597295

Charon, R. (2001b, Jan 2). Narrative medicine: form, function, and ethics. *Annals of Internal Medicine, 134*(1), 83–87. http://dx.doi.org/10.7326/0003-4819-134-1-200101020-00024 Medline:11187429

Charon, R. (2006). *Narrative medicine: Honoring the stories of illness.* New York: Oxford University Press.

Chatman, S.B. (2000). Point of view. In M. McQuillan (Ed.), *The narrative reader* (pp. 96–98). London: Routledge.

DasGupta, S. (2006). Being John Doe Malkovich: Truth, imagination, and story in medicine. *Literature and Medicine, 25*(2), 439–462. http://dx.doi.org/10.1353/lm.2007.0003

Donohoe, M.T. (2009). Stories and society: Using literature to teach medical students about public health and social justice. *International Journal of the Creative Arts in Interdisciplinary Practice, 8.*

Engel, S. (1995). *The stories children tell: Making sense of the narratives of childhood.* New York: W.H. Freeman and Company.

Engel, S. (2005). *Real kids: Creating meaning in everyday life.* Cambridge, MA: Harvard University Press.

Forster, E.M. (1927). *Aspects of the novel.* San Diego: Harcourt, Inc.

Fox, M. (1997). Is there life after Foucault? Texts, frames, and differends. In A. Petersen & R. Bunton (Eds.), *Foucault, health, and medicine* (pp. 31–50). New York: Routledge.

Goldhagen, J. (2005, Apr). Integrating pediatrics and public health. *Pediatrics, 115*(4 Suppl), 1202–1208. http://dx.doi.org/10.1542/peds.2004-2825U Medline:15821311

Hay, E. (2000). *A student of weather.* Toronto: McClelland & Stewart.

Hildick, E.W. (1971). *Children and fiction: A critical study of the artistic and psychological factors involved in writing fiction for and about children.* New York: World Publishing Company.

Jung, C.G. (1963). The psychology of the child archetype. In C.G. Jung & C. Kerenyi (Eds.), *Essays on a science of mythology: The myths of the divine child and the divine maiden* (Rev. ed, pp. 70–98). (R.F.C. Hull, Trans.). New York: Harper & Row.

Little, M. (2003). Does reading poetry make you a better clinician? In I. Kerridge, C. Jordens, & E. Sayers (Eds.), *Restoring humane values to medicine: A Miles Little reader* (pp. 45–48). Annandale, NSW, Australia: Desert Pea Press.

Manworren, R.C., & Woodring, B. (1998, Nov–Dec). Evaluating children's literature as a source for patient education. *Pediatric Nursing, 24*(6), 548–553. Medline:10085997

Mendelsohn, J.S., Quinn, M.T., & McNabb, W.L. (1999, Feb). Interview strategies commonly used by pediatricians. *Archives of Pediatrics & Adolescent Medicine, 153*(2), 154–157. http://dx.doi.org/10.1001/archpedi.153.2.154 Medline:9988245

Montgomery, L.M. (1983). *Anne of Green Gables.* Toronto: Seal Books. [1908].

Perrin, E.C., & Starr, S. (2000, Apr). Addressing common pediatric concerns through children's books. *Pediatrics in Review, 21*(4), 130–138. http://dx.doi.org/10.1542/pir.21-4-130 Medline:10756176

Rapezzi, C., Ferrari, R., & Branzi, A. (2005, Dec 24). White coats and fingerprints: diagnostic reasoning in medicine and investigative methods of fictional detectives. *BMJ (Clinical Research Ed.), 331*(7531), 1491–1494. http://dx.doi.org/10.1136/bmj.331.7531.1491 Medline:16373725

Siourbas, H. (2003). L.M. Montgomery: Canon or cultural capital? In A. Hudson & S. Cooper (Eds.), *Windows and words: A look at Canadian children's literature in English* (pp. 131–141). Ottawa: University of Ottawa Press.

Smith, B.H. (1980). Narrative versions, narrative theories. *Critical Inquiry, 7*(1), 213–236. http://dx.doi.org/10.1086/448097

Wolraich, M.L., Wolraich, M., Dworkin, P.H., Drotar, D.D., & Perrin, E.C. (2008). *Developmental-behavioral pediatrics: Evidence and practice.* Philadelphia: Mosby.

Lifelines

The Healing Arts Program, St. Paul's Hospital, Saskatoon, Saskatchewan

Marlessa Wesolowski and Christopher Cooper

The Healing Arts Program at St. Paul's Hospital is supported through generous donations to the St. Paul's Hospital Foundation. It was developed in collaboration between the hospital's Mission Office, within which the Artist in Residence (AIR) resides, and the hospital's

MOM
Your love is Family.
Your Love is in all of us.
Your heart is part of us.
We will be Strong.
Now Fly, Fly.
Fly Like a Angel
We All love you.
MOM.
Love You
Baby Girl
Mom

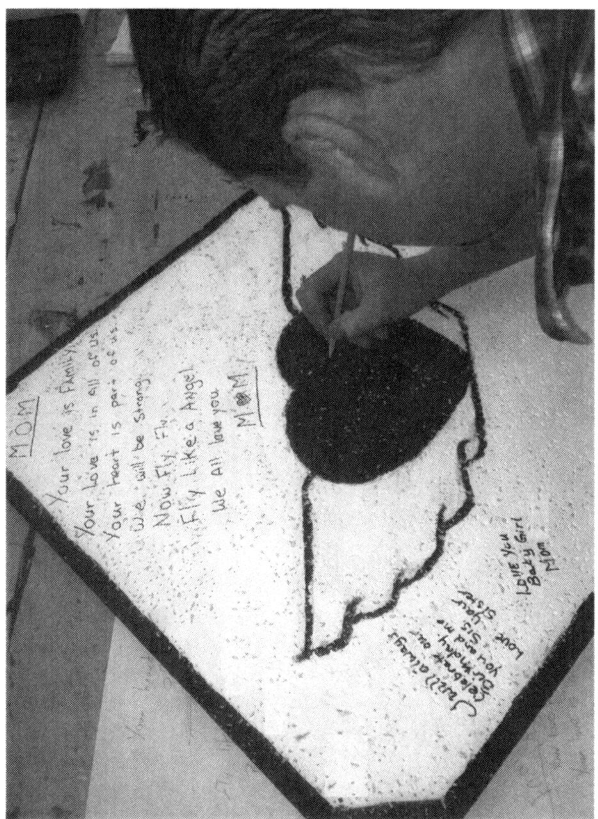

Figure L.2 "Angel Wings"; photo by Marlessa Wesolowski

Volunteer Workforce Department to enhance whole-person care for individual and community health. The AIR integrates the positive benefits of creativity into a health care setting using an approach of arts-based unconditional positive regard with diverse arts activities.

The purpose of the program is to enhance the compassionate, holistic concept of care the hospital provides. The AIR was introduced at St. Paul's Hospital in 2005 in response to an identified need for a complementary non-medical method to encourage therapeutic processes through creativity and using an arts-based methodology. The hemodialysis unit, for example, understands that, for a patient in a technically driven health care system, increased positive self-concept is desired but not easily attainable. As a regular part of their lives, hemodialysis patients have medical procedures three times a week at four hours per treatment. For many of these patients much of their previous lifestyle is no longer accessible to them. The AIR practices a method that cultivates presence and concentrates primarily on processes associated with concepts of self in a healing environment. Presence is a fundamental principle and is considered by many humanistic theorists to be central to effecting meaningful change. The AIR operates on the principle that an increased sense of well-being contributes to healing goals.

SECTION 4

THE CREATIVE ARTS IN ACTION FOR CHANGE IN HEALTH

13

Arts-Based Inquiry and a Clinician Educator's Journey of Discovery

Louise Younie, GP

Medical-student learning has been dominated by depersonalized disease-based knowledge acquisition. Students are trained with the skills to diagnose and treat disease. I do not contest the value of knowledge- and skills-based learning, but in this chapter I would like to invite extension of the knowledge(s) we consider relevant for future doctors and how medical-student engagement with the arts might broaden practitioner epistemology. Engagement in arts-based inquiry opens other dimensions of knowing. Personal creative–reflective knowledge production through engaging with the more metaphorical, poetic and symbolic language of the arts can offer deepened reflection and insight. Student production of creative–reflective texts within any of the arts-based media invites voice, liminality, evocation, emotion and perspective, thereby extending interpersonal and practice-based learning. This interpersonal and holistic approach to practitioner development may complement the increasing competency-based approach being adopted at medical schools (Kuper, 2006). In contrast to arts-based inquiry, which nurtures interconnected and values-based knowing, a competency-based approach builds on a behaviourist framework, which breaks clinical work into "small discrete tasks" and potentially ignores the "complex nature of situations in the real world" (Leung, 2002, p. 693).

Drawing on the concept of arts-based inquiry in the research field, arts-based inquiry in medical education might be described as "the … making of artistic expressions … as a primary way of understanding and examining experience" (McNiff, 2008, p. 29). To explore this relatively new field of arts-based inquiry, I draw on the literature as well as my work as clinician and educator, illustrating with examples that have arisen over the last 10 years of engaging students in this field of learning. I begin by considering the context for the emergence of arts-based inquiry in medical education as well as within my own sphere of work. The practical dimension of facilitating arts-based inquiry will be explored through two case studies reviewing delivery, assessment and evaluation. This section will be followed by consideration of learning through the arts and the potential for practice or practitioner development.

Emergence of Arts-Based Inquiry in Medical Education

Arts-based inquiry expands the concept of medical humanities, taking medical students beyond being consumers of the artistic creation of others to producing their own creative–reflective texts. This mode of education moves away from the more traditional "transmissive" approach to learning, instead inviting students into a "transformative, dialogical, and reciprocal encounter" (Milligan & Woodley, 2009, p. 134). It is not so much about putting learning into students as drawing it out through collaborative reflective spaces where practice and context can be explored beyond the purely cognitive realm—embracing also the affective, experiential and existential (Kumagai, 2012).

To contextualize arts-based inquiry within medical education I must briefly consider the evolution of the field of medical humanities. The term *medical humanities* has been variously defined as lists of subjects, domains of practice (medical education, arts for health, etc.) and lines of inquiry (Brody, 2011; Evans, 2008). The medical humanities have been described within American medical schools since the 1970s (Charon et al., 1995) and been increasingly popular in the United Kingdom and internationally over the last 15 to 20 years (Lazarus & Rosslyn, 2003). Surveys have shown that medical-student curricula are increasingly engaging with the spectrum of the arts; for example, in 2002 Rodenhauser, Strickland and Gambala (2004) conducted a survey that showed more than half of the respondents from medical schools in the United States used the arts in a learning activity (Kumagai, 2012). In 2003–2004, there was at least one required medical humanities course in 88 out of 125 American medical schools and an elective course offered at 55 (Kuper, 2006). This has been mirrored by the increasing numbers of medical humanities publications in high-impact medical journals (e.g., *Lancet, BMJ*) and medical-education journals *(Medical Education, Academic Medicine)* (Kuper, 2006). Despite such interest, the medical humanities remain a marginalized field (Gordon, 2005), often delivered as additive courses rather than integrated into the core curriculum (Evans & Greaves, 1999), "classified as merely enrichment opportunities" rather than "integral components of health care instruction" (Friedman, 2002, p. 320). Much pedagogical writing has been dedicated to justifying the arts and humanities within medical education (Brody, 2011; Kuper, 2006), yet more work is needed in terms of theoretical underpinning and evidence of changed practice (Gordon, 2005). Drawing on my own qualitative research (Younie, 2006, 2011) and experience in the field, I seek to contribute student and clinician perspectives, offer qualitative evidence of changed thinking (which may lead to changed practice) and develop theoretical understanding of the contributions arts-based inquiry makes to medical education.

Over time we have made progress in the practical delivery of the medical humanities in the undergraduate curriculum. At inception, the medical humanities tended to be predominantly literary (Kuper, 2006; Evans, 2008) and often involved engagement in poetry or narratives written by others. Although as far back as 1995 there are examples of student engagement in creative–reflective writing to help develop their understanding of patient encounters (Charon et al., 1995), offering students the spectrum of the arts for reflection on themselves, their experiences and their context or to explore practice is a much more recent phenomenon. This may be due to the greater gap from written language to interpretive and embodied communication through, for example, the performing and visual arts.

There are relatively few examples in the literature of medical student engagement with the creative process through the arts. Examples include facilitation of arts-based inquiry courses through artist-led electives (de la Croix, Rose, Wildig & Willson, 2011; Dumitriu, 2009), artist–clinician collaborations (Gull, 2005; Weller, 2002; Younie, 2013) and medical-educator innovations (Thompson, Lamont-Robinson & Younie, 2010; Kumagai, 2012; LoFaso, Breckman, Capello, Demopoulos & Adelman, 2010). The learning often relates to development of broadened understanding and perspectives. Examples include engaging with visual installation work for communicating ideas around the practice of medicine (Dumitriu, 2009), creative textual production to foster a patient-centred and reflective approach (Kumagai, 2012) or the use of art to express and extend learning from encounters with patients suffering chronic illness (LoFaso et al., 2010)

Emergence of Arts-Based Inquiry in My Educational Practice

> "... listen to the world and so allow changes to take place"
>
> —*H.J.M. Nouwen (1998, p. 52)*

My journey into arts-based inquiry as an educator began in response to encountering patients in practice and there finding a growing sense of the inadequacy of the medical toolkit of diagnosis and management. As I entered the family-practice setting, my patients as my teachers, with their complex needs and array of suffering, began to draw out of me new ways of doctoring. Engaging with patient suffering takes us beyond the physical, into the social, emotional and existential realms, beyond the biomedical into the biographical where the "parameters are metaphysical: hope, despair, guilt, uncertainty and fear" (Sweeney, 2005, p. 224). Here the medical toolkit offers not the way of engaging with or alleviating patient suffering but *one* way, a one-dimensional tool for three-dimensional problems. A complementary strand of my practice needing attention was the doctor as therapeutic agent, where presence, listening, silence and journeying with the patient all reside.

The question that challenged me, as a newly qualified GP and novice in education, was how to facilitate future doctor communication of their science with patients in healing and therapeutic ways. I realized that different ways *to* knowing (Seeley, 2011) were necessary in this realm of therapeutic agency. While acquiring the knowledge needed to diagnose and treat disease might be an intellectual pursuit, development of interpersonal and practice-based understanding is a more personal, embodied and applied endeavour. This dimension of future practice cannot be taught so much as encouraged and facilitated. Seeking to create extended reflective spaces for exploratory and transformative work led me into engagement with the arts. The artistry on my part has been as "artist of the invisible," gardening to create these potentially transformative spaces (Seeley, 2011). In the following sections I will explore two different approaches to facilitating student arts-based inquiry, one university based and the other clinical. Another local example pioneered by Dr. Trevor Thompson has been discussed elsewhere (Thompson et al., 2010).

Creative Arts Student-Selected Components (SSC)

> ... we have recently been taught about the complexities of the visual pathway: the journey from the retinal ganglion cells, through the lateral geniculate nucleus and into the occipital lobe; yet it is my participation in courses such as the SSC in Creative Arts and doing a creative piece for our GP Placement last year, that has encouraged me to remember that this pathway is so much more than an anatomical tract. For people with visual impairments, their raised intraocular pressure is isolation. The degeneration of their macular is never being able to see their grandchildren's faces. And it is these consequences that distress and worry the patient, not the underlying pathological defect. This course has emphasized to me the importance of seeing past the diagnosis and focusing instead on the patient ...
>
> —*Katherine Turner, post-course SSC reflection, 2011*

My first step toward experiential and creative learning for medical students involved seeking out spaces and places in the curriculum where courses might be added or developed. Initially, after gaining funding, I created an optional Student-Selected Component (SSC), which involved eight co-facilitated workshop sessions with myself as clinical bridge and collaborating with a variety of arts for health or arts-therapy practitioners. This approach differs from what has been reported in the literature in two ways: by focusing on the therapeutic dimension of the arts for health and because of the presence of both clinician and arts-based facilitator in the sessions (for comparison see Dumitriu, 2009; Weller, 2002; Gull, 2005; de la Croix et al., 2011). Small groups (usually 7 to 13) of self-selecting second-year students have engaged with this experiential–reflective course annually since 2004. Sessions focus on diverse areas such as music therapy, art therapy, art for health, creative writing, drama, photography and film. Students hear about ways of engaging patients therapeutically with the arts and experience some of the methods for themselves. Some sessions involve sharing patient-produced creative texts such as drawing, painting and songwriting.

Assessment

Assessment has three parts to represent different aspects of learning in the course, including personal, propositional (Higgs & Titchen, 2000) and presentational knowing (meaning-making through symbol and imagery) (Heron & Reason, 1997). Assessment tasks are relatively open ended and include a reflective journal (which is assessed for depth of reflection rather than content), a referenced essay linking art and science (past titles include "Poetry as Therapy," "The Art of Medicine," "The Artist and His Illness," etc.) and the production of a creative–reflective text.

Regarding the reflective journaling, students are provided with a choice of different-shaped and -coloured reflective journals in the first session and are encouraged not just to write but to sketch, paint, use collage and so on as they consider their experiences of each session. Students sometimes find or create their own journals or means of collecting their reflections. One student produced his reflective journal electronically, using a series of found images to accompany his reflective writing. He used the image of two frightened infants in a butcher shop with the caption "James and I fretting before the session … I wasn't that keen on showing off my lack of drawing skills in front of everyone …" (2010; note that student name has been changed). The next image is of a cat sunbathing on a deckchair and the note "How relaxed I was after the session got underway."

The creative–reflective text part of the assessment has been met by student engagement in a variety of media such as painting, photography, film, poetry, music and even baking. Students have embraced a wide spectrum of themes from medical to more personal dimensions. The following example was inspired by two local patient texts seen in this course, one of which spoke of an idea in a Cuban novel of having "two hearts. One that we keep for ourselves, the other that we give away."

> There was a particular painting by a patient that consistently caught my eye. It was of a small, dark explosion in the corner with radiating hues of blues, yellows and browns that appeared to signify life going on around the little outburst, which was the patient themselves. I took inspiration from this painting and wanted mine to reflect the style of that patient's (hence the explosive nature of my background) so that I was, in a way connecting with them. Even though I have never met them, I feel as though their painting gives me just the slightest of insights into their life, and I respect them immensely for being willing to try to express their situation, and allowing me to have just the smallest of peeks into their experiences of life …
>
> —*Medical student, Sophie Swinhoe, 2011*

Sophie's reflection goes on to explore at depth the imagery and symbolism in her work and the way it meaningfully relates to her professional work with patients. I am struck by Sophie's attention to the patient narrative and imagery. It is this kind of attention to the actual patient in the consultation that I seek to encourage.

Course Evaluation

Evaluation takes place in qualitative fashion through pre- and post-course questionnaires and a final focus group. I also learn a great deal about the students' experience of the course through their dialogue in the sessions and their reflective journals. It could be argued that

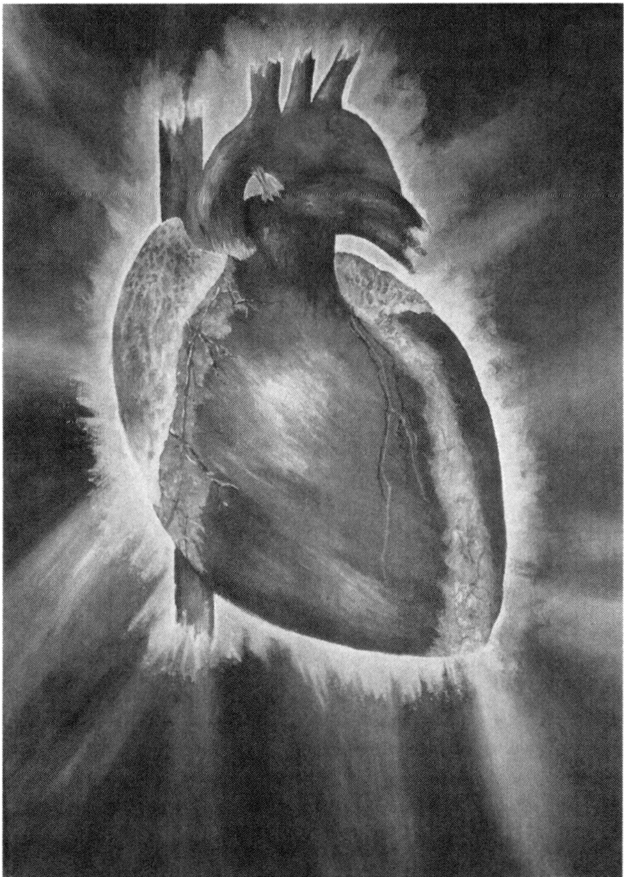

Figure 13.1 Heart painting by Sophie Swinhoe

these modes of evaluation might limit students' negative critique of the course, yet the course ethos is to express varied ideas and opinions, and students have, over the years, noted at least some issues that have arisen.

The SSC Student Experience

According to their pre-course questionnaires, most students enroll in this course because of their interest in extended ways of encouraging health for future patients. They also look forward to opportunities for their own creative expression (although some, as expressed above, are nervous). Many are surprised, however, at the journey they end up taking through the creative–reflective and collaborative process (Younie, 2006). One student wrote,

> I've really enjoyed the opportunity to participate in the course and as well as learning a lot about a range of therapy options, it has been good for learning a lot about ourselves ... (2005)

Surprising to me has been that, despite the different co-facilitators and different groups of students each year, some very similar themes arise across our group dialogue, the students' reflective journals, focus groups and interviews (Younie, 2006). These themes relate to the learning environment and to their learning.

Learning in this course differs from learning in much of the rest of the curriculum, being experiential, reflective, collaborative and emergent. The learning environment is described by students as a "breath of fresh air" and an opportunity to "think again." Students are struck by the interpretive environment, not having to come up with the "right answer." They notice in sharing their divergent perspectives that their learning is enhanced.

> The creative process feels a bit like a window to life—a sense of thought explosions—and it has been great to have an opportunity to let these thoughts grow in an open understanding space.
>
> I have already seen a change in how I think and question things, just from one session of creative arts. I have spoken to a couple of members of the group about this and asked if they have seen any change in their thought process ... like me they have said that they have began noticing what previously stayed unnoticed and have given thought to subjects that they have never previously considered. (2011)

Another theme relating to the learning environment is the quality of dialogue and sharing among peers.

> I remember writing lots that I felt privileged in the diary ... because you don't usually get to see that side of people and I think it's a real honor when people decide that they feel comfortable enough or trust the group or you enough that they can open up like that ... (2005)

Students often put this trust down to the group being self-selected and open, but also I believe that collaborative risk-taking spaces are opened up through the very act of creative expression and sharing.

> ... the feeling in the room was invigorating. How electric. A mixture of nervousness of self-expression in front of peers; awe at one another's craft, gratitude towards each other ... personal thoughts and positive feedback ... laughter seems to make it all the more healthy ... (2011)

One student reflecting on this during the first session talked of not being able to be creative without putting something of oneself into the work and that this was potentially exposing and certainly unfamiliar within the context of medical education.

Students note that the course was "emotionally quite hard work" and talk about coming away from some of the sessions feeling "drained and thoughtful": one student remarked, "I was surprised how many of the group produced very emotional pieces. Maybe this was a reflection of the session, that the pieces of work we had observed were very meaningful" (2005). The emotional dimension is encountered through patient narratives of suffering, for example, through song or imagery as well as some student sharing of their own narratives. This quotation relates to dialogue resulting after a personal narrative shared around death:

> ... we scratched the surface of the huge dark entity, paying enough attention to it ... not to have felt awkward or uncomfortable but to have felt as if we were making progress together on a deeper level, organic and fluid, not contrived ... (2011)

Although the emotions were at times challenging, many students embrace the emotional dimension and value this opportunity for shared exploration of what will be a dimension of their future practice (Younie, 2006): "I think those were the sessions I gained the most out of although they were the heaviest" (2005). Still, some discomfort has been expressed by three students over the years. One student proposed more preparation before potentially emotional sessions—for example, when an artist told his life story with lymphoma through his paintings. One student mentioned using humour to lighten the sometimes heavy atmosphere, and another recognized the proximity of the group work at times to a "therapy group session." Careful facilitation is therefore necessary, despite that we recognize the value of exploring these spaces before encountering them in clinical practice.

Student Learning

> ... but we weren't learning. And yet I have learnt so much in the course without necessarily learning anything. We were thinking. The long pauses and wide open questions which were so often part of the session seemed to have taught us ... to interpret things and make connections ... (2011)

Students talk about learning life-long lessons or not being sure at all of what they have learned. Learning has been described on the level of "revelation" involving personal insight and learning about themselves as well as becoming more aware of the "Other" and the intersubjectivity of interpersonal communication:

> I think that today demonstrated to me the intricacies of human experience ... that everyone is very different and that behind any façade there lies a wealth of individual thoughts and experiences. (2005)

Meeting the patient as a person is another key theme noted by students in this course:

> One of the main lessons of this SSC for me at least, was about the complex nature of patients and the impossibilities of really knowing them or understanding them, particularly in a GPs limited time. Despite this impossibility, the course has encouraged the belief that just trying to understand patients better and look at them more holistically has a lot of benefits. … I have been encouraged … to meet each patient as a person, and to … help them, not just treat them.
>
> … these thoughts about the complexity of patients … often skipped over in medical school … are reflected in my final reflexive text. I have tried to represent this beauty and complexity as fantastic images and bright colors and to show that it is inextricably linked to the other aspects of medicine in the form of the picture.
>
> —*Medical student, Stephanie Greenwald, 2012*

Students also engage with their own personhood and experiences. It is not unusual for students to write a poem or share a photograph capturing struggles they face as medical students, often resulting in group dialogue, shared perspectives and relief.

Challenges

Challenges I faced as course organizer of this kind of learning included finding funding for this work, space in the curriculum and arts-based co-facilitators to collaborate with. Students are self-selecting and therefore usually very open to the different ideas and educational environment they face. For the facilitator, being confident in facilitating and maintaining a safe transformative space is also central.

First-Year GP Placement

A different way of inviting students into arts-based inquiry learning exists within clinical placements. The two examples found in the literature related to community placements, as does my own experience. Kumagai (2012) invites first-year students in small groups to explore their different experiences of the patient encounter. In their groups they choose a creative medium to communicate "themes, emotions or perspectives" (p. 1139) and these projects are presented to their peers. LoFaso, Breckman, Capello, Demopoulos and Adelman (2010) report on multi-disciplinary faculty working with third- and fourth-year medical students who are invited to share found or original art to express reactions and thoughts relating to home visits they have made. My own experience, as course organizer for a first-year community placement in general practice (2002–2010), differs from these examples in that individual students were invited to produce original creative–reflective texts to capture patients' lived experience or the students' lived experience in encounters with the patient. Front-line clinicians running the placements were asked to both respond to and formatively grade the student work.

Assessment originally involved a reflective essay based on a chosen home-visit encounter with a patient. In 2004, I introduced the option of producing a creative–reflective text instead of the essay format. That year I received 12 pieces of creative writing from a cohort of 250. In following years I offered some encouragement to explore the creative process in my course introductory lecture and shared some of the high-quality student texts produced in the previous year. The result was that medical students continued to stretch this educational space and diversified in their creative explorations to produce paintings, photography, dance and musical compositions, sculpture and more. By 2010, 78% of the year were choosing the creative–reflective option, often producing high-quality aesthetic and reflective texts. According to post-course questionnaires (Younie, 2011), reasons for student effort and engagement in this formative assessment, which does not count toward their ranking, include their gratitude at the openness and generosity of patients offering their lived experiences, encouragement by their GP tutor, the introductory lecture and this course being a rare opportunity within the curriculum for interpretation and exploration of the more personal dimension of medical practice. The small-group context (two or three students) placed with each GP may also be facilitative.

One of the highlights for me, as an educator inviting students to engage with arts-based inquiry in this course, has been the increasing expression of student voice and personal knowing within their reflective texts. There has been movement from more of a written report with some reflection added toward an approach that is independent, creative and critical (Milligan & Woodley, 2009) as evidenced in the following two excerpts. In the first example, the first-year student positions herself as neophyte medical trainee, the metaphorical blank canvas, exploring her feelings and what the patient might be thinking.

Paint my canvas

I am a canvas,
As blank as can be,
Inexperienced in suffering,
Ill-health still a mystery to me,
I sit waiting for your paintbrush,

For the colours to unveil,
I sit, I wait ...

Around you I am helpless.
Around you I feel ashamed.
Ashamed of my youth,
My energy and smile,
Ashamed to giggle or joke for a while,
I want to understand you,
See through your waning smile.

Will you let me in?
Unlock your past,
And let me into your present,
You have so much to offer,
I won't let it go to waste.
My nonchalance and ignorance,
I'm sure is all you see,
But I'm willing and I'm waiting,
I sit, I wait.

Then at once,
Your story awakens me,
Sends shivers up my spine,
I am left floundering,
Choked up.
For reasons I cannot describe,
Your calm, quiet voice sits screaming,
"Wake up and welcome to life" ...

—Georgina Maguire, 2010

The next example is of a student writing from the perspective of a patient with a chronic illness.

I was ... relieved to finally have a diagnosis, at last someone recognizing that there was something actually wrong with me and that I wasn't just some weirdo who was imagining things. It had taken them over a year to figure it out ... All the time I had doctors brushing it aside; "oh it's probably nothing more than such and such" they said dismissively like I didn't know what I was feeling in my own body.

Meanwhile I kept falling over for no apparent reason, my leg felt shorter to me than it actually was so I was always stumbling. It was like when you reach the bottom of some stairs and don't realize till you put your foot out for the next step which isn't there ...

... Those students looked so young, still it's nice to talk to them that way, somewhere down the line at those medical schools I reckon they learn to stop listening. Part of the process I guess, like learning how to handle blood and guts and stuff. Of course I don't mean just hearing what I'm saying; they have to do that to know what's wrong. I mean listening, taking the time to hear the worry in my voice and giving some comfort and confirmation that it's not just all in my head. Perhaps I've just had bad experiences, but I've had enough of them ...

—*George Wellby, 2010*

These texts highlight two key areas of interpersonal development and reflection that are potentially nurtured through arts-based inquiry, namely reflexivity and narrative humility (Younie, 2011). By reflexivity I mean awareness of how our internal framework affects our view and interpretation of the world, and by narrative humility I mean the students' ability to engage insightfully and compassionately with patient narratives (DasGupta, 2008). Of course, reflection without engagement with the language of the arts could facilitate a degree of such learning, but my experience suggests that, as in these examples, imaginatively considering another's perspective or metaphorical consideration of oneself in context may go further to encourage extension of horizons. Such development of understanding of "self" and "Other" are the building blocks for development of empathy (Clark, 2000) and patient-centred practice (Campion, Foulkes, Neighbour, Tate & Membership of the Royal College of General Practitioners, 2002).

Challenges

Challenges to the introduction of arts-based inquiry into clinical placements include student cynicism, faculty cynicism, grading, confidentiality in sharing of patient stories and finding capacity to develop such options within the time, financial and curricular constraints.

Student cynicism, an issue noted in other medical-humanities contexts (Shapiro, Coulehan, Wear & Montello, 2009), has not really been a problem given the safety valve of the creative–reflective text being optional. Other safety valves in this kind of work include inviting the students to work in small groups on a creative text (Kumagai, 2012) or allowing students to either produce original art or to use found art (LoFaso et al., 2010). Regarding faculty cynicism, validating an arts-based inquiry assessment both with clinicians and at the university has taken some effort. Feedback about the arts-based inquiry option was sought annually from the front-line general practitioner (GP) tutors engaging with the student work. Although many were surprised and impressed with what the students were capable of expressing, noting the depth of student "emotional and empathic response[s]," some felt like a creative–reflective text was an easy option, "hardly a rigorous test of ability" (Younie, 2011). Regarding the challenge of marking this work, criteria developed (by me and artist Dr. Catherine Lamont-Robinson) of impact, perception, reflection and aesthetics were welcomed. However, some GPs continued to find the marking difficult due to, for example, perceived subjectivity of such work, considering themselves not creative and feeling that constructive criticism might be taken more personally than with a traditional essay (Younie, 2011). Growing acceptance of this educational approach is illustrated, however, through increasing student and therefore GP-tutor engagement and also commendation by the General Medical Council on their last medical school appraisal visit to the University of Bristol (2009).

A further issue is that of confidentiality. Both Kumagai (2012) and LoFaso, Breckman, Capello, Demopoulos and Adelman (2010) have focused on general themes and learning points arising rather than an in-depth exploration of the patient narrative. The advantage with this approach is that it is less personal, and so for Kumagai it is possible to showcase the student work inviting patient volunteers as well as faculty and students to an evening event. Although we have instances where GPs show student work to the patient, this is done carefully and within the context of the GP surgery and a trusting GP–patient relationship.

A final challenge to mention as clinician-educator is the costliness of this work, not so much financially (although this can be a limiting factor) but instead in terms of hours laid down, investment of self and different paradigms spanned. Yet the reward is great. I learn from the patients' lived experience through the eyes of the students. The evocative work of the students invites me to see the clinical world afresh, inhabiting as they do a "liminal" space between lay person and clinician, being "between two conditions, yet fully inhabiting neither" (Elliott, 2011, p. 96).

Learning Spaces Opened Through the Arts

I have sought to illustrate the potential for learning when arts-based reflective spaces are opened up to medical students. Particular to such learning spaces are the new vocabularies and languages of expression, the opportunities for imaginative engagement with other perspectives, group learning and sharing of personal perspective and interpretation, group engagement with the creative process, and personal and collaborative creative–reflective knowledge production. These learning opportunities seem to invite a more holistic engagement in the complexity of practice.

The arts invite new vocabularies of colour, form, rhythm, silence, metaphor and symbolism. Through these languages rich engagement with the world of emotion, meaning-making, ambiguity and not knowing is possible (Elliott, 2011). Such are domains of thinking and being, unusual within the medical curriculum, yet commonly part of daily clinical practice.

Extension of horizons may be encouraged through imaginative engagement with a different position—that of patient or caregiver, for example—to consider what another might see or experience. Where group dialogue is employed around student texts, it offers multiple perspectives and ways of seeing that might further extend learning from an experience (LoFaso et al., 2010; Charon & Hermann, 2012). Further, educator interest in the student perspective and lived experience (rather than just technical knowledge and skills) may encourage students to be likewise interested in their future patients' lived experiences.

Group engagement in the silent active creative process, or "flow" (Csikszentmihalyi, 1990), offers students a different way of being with each other, inviting them to experience meaningful spaces without words. Engagement in the creative process itself invites exploration and reworking of observations and insights, thereby slowing down perception and offering the time to really look (Eisner, 2002). As Comete-Sponville (2005) remarks, "All arts are like mirrors in which Man learns and recognizes something of himself of which he was unaware" (p. 100). Although there is evidence within the student work for many of the above ideas, it is also important to note that the arts are purely a vehicle for this work. This means that they can be used in the above ways to enhance learning from practice and interpersonal encounters; however, they can also be used to perpetuate limited ways of seeing and understanding others or to be engaged with as an easy option or without the aesthetic depth of accompanying meaning-making.

Extending Ways of Knowing

For both educators (Kumagai, 2012) and researchers (Elliott, 2011; Seeley, 2011), participatory engagement with the arts is seen to extend or potentially to facilitate different, more holistic ways of knowing. Kumagai (2012) focuses on the development of understanding in the realm of "tacit knowledge" (Polanyi, 1967) gained through human interactions. Elliott (2011) and Seeley (2011) consider the embodied and holistic dimension of lived experience elucidated through arts-based methods, allowing entry to the "wholeness of experience" (Elliott, 2011, p. 102) or being "pulled towards a whole human knowing" (Seeley, 2011, p. 85). In contrast, word-based methods have been criticized for limiting "the extent to which researchers can explore the multiple ways in which human experiences are enacted and understood" (Liamputtong & Rumbold, 2008, p. 15).

Relating this to the educational context, I would like to suggest that arts-based inquiry could work to draw out the wholeness of student experience more fully in practice, i.e., practice-based learning, a dimension of learning under-represented in the undergraduate curriculum (Shapiro et al., 2009), which links with Schön's (1983) "professional artistry" or Higgs and Titchen's (2000) "professional craft knowledge." This is the learning that takes place in encounter with the complexity, uncertainty and interpersonal human dimension of clinical practice. McIntosh (2010) suggests that such learning is not inevitable, practitioners/future practitioners have the choice "to sleepwalk through the experience and gain nothing new from it; or to engage with it in order to understand it and our self better through it" (p. 28).

NOTE

I would like to thank both the arts-based facilitators with whom I have worked over the years and the students who have engaged with this arts-based inquiry process and have shared their creative work and perspectives.

REFERENCES

Brody, H. (2011, Mar). Defining the medical humanities: three conceptions and three narratives. *Journal of Medical Humanities, 32*(1), 1–7. http://dx.doi.org/10.1007/s10912-009-9094-4 Medline:19936898

Campion, P., Foulkes, J., Neighbour, R., Tate, P., & Membership of the Royal College of General Practitioners. (2002, Sep 28). Patient centredness in the MRCGP video examination: analysis of large cohort. *BMJ (Clinical Research Ed.), 325*(7366), 691–692. http://dx.doi.org/10.1136/bmj.325.7366.691 Medline:12351363

Charon, R., Banks, J.T., Connelly, J.E., et al. (1995, Apr 15). Literature and medicine: contributions to clinical practice. *Annals of Internal Medicine, 122*(8), 599–606. http://dx.doi.org/10.7326/0003-4819-122-8-199504150-00008 Medline:7887555

Charon, R., & Hermann, N. (2012, Jan). Commentary: a sense of story, or why teach reflective writing? *Academic Medicine, 87*(1), 5–7. http://dx.doi.org/10.1097/ACM.0b013e31823a59c7 Medline:22201631

Clark, J.L. (2000). *Beyond empathy: An ethnographic approach to cross-cultural social work practice.* Toronto: Faculty of Social Work, University of Toronto.

Comete-Sponville, A. (2005). *The little book of philosophy.* London: Vintage.

Csikszentmihalyi, M. (1990). *Flow: The psychology of optimal experience.* New York: Harper and Row.

DasGupta, S. (2008, Mar 22). Narrative humility. *Lancet, 371*(9617), 980–981. http://dx.doi.org/10.1016/S0140-6736(08)60440-7 Medline:18363204

de la Croix, A., Rose, C., Wildig, E., & Willson, S. (2011, Nov). Arts-based learning in medical education: the students' perspective. *Medical Education, 45*(11), 1090–1100. http://dx.doi.org/10.1111/j.1365-2923.2011.04060.x Medline:21988624

Dumitriu, A. (2009). Creative communication for medical students: Using installation and performance art to communicate ideas about medicine. *The Academy Subject Centre for Medicine, Dentistry and Veterinary Medicine Newsletter* 01, 20, 23–25.

Eisner, E. (2002). *The arts and the creation of mind.* Virginia: R.R. Donnelley & Sons.

Elliott, B. (2011). Arts-based and narrative inquiry in liminal experience reveal platforming as basic social psychological process. *Arts in Psychotherapy, 38*(2), 96–103. http://dx.doi.org/10.1016/j.aip.2011.01.001

Evans, H.M. (2008, Mar). Affirming the existential within medicine: medical humanities, governance, and imaginative understanding. *Journal of Medical Humanities, 29*(1), 55–59. http://dx.doi.org/10.1007/s10912-007-9051-z Medline:18058207

Evans, M., & Greaves, D. (1999, Nov 6). Exploring the medical humanities. *BMJ (Clinical Research Ed.), 319*(7219), 1216–1216. http://dx.doi.org/10.1136/bmj.319.7219.1216 Medline:10550065

Friedman, L.D. (2002, Apr). The precarious position of the medical humanities in the medical school curriculum. *Academic Medicine, 77*(4), 320–322. http://dx.doi.org/10.1097/00001888-200204000-00011 Medline:11953297

Gordon, J. (2005). Not everything that counts can be counted. *Medical Education, 39*(6), 551–554. http://dx.doi.org/10.1111/j.1365-2929.2005.02201.x

Gull, S. (2005). Life drawing in undergraduate clinical attachments. *The Academy Subject Centre for Medicine. Dentistry and Veterinary Medicine Newsletter, 01*, 8–9.

Heron, J., & Reason, P. (1997). A participative inquiry paradigm. *Qualitative Inquiry, 3*(3), 274–294. http://dx.doi.org/10.1177/107780049700300302

Higgs, J., & Titchen, A. (2000). Knowledge and reasoning. In J. Higgs & M. Jones (Eds.), *Clinical reasoning in the health professions* (pp. 23–32). Oxford: Butterworth-Heinemann.

Kumagai, A.K. (2012, Aug). Perspective: acts of interpretation: a philosophical approach to using creative arts in medical education. *Academic Medicine, 87*(8), 1138–1144. http://dx.doi.org/10.1097/ACM.0b013e31825d0fd7 Medline:22722358

Kuper, A. (2006, Oct). Literature and medicine: A problem of assessment. *Academic Medicine, 81*(10 Suppl), S128–S137. http://dx.doi.org/10.1097/00001888-200610001-00032 Medline:17001123

Lazarus, P.A., & Rosslyn, F.M. (2003, Jun). The Arts in Medicine: setting up and evaluating a new special study module at Leicester Warwick Medical School. *Medical Education, 37*(6), 553–559. http://dx.doi.org/10.1046/j.1365-2923.2003.01537.x Medline:12787379

Leung, W.C. (2002). Learning in practice: Competency-based medical training [review]. *BMJ (Clinical Research Ed.), 325*, 693–695. http://dx.doi.org/10.1136/bmj.325.7366.693 Medline:12351364

Liamputtong, P. & Rumbold, J. (Eds.). (2008). *Knowing differently: Arts-based and collaborative research methods.* New York: Nova Science Publishers.

LoFaso, V.M., Breckman, R., Capello, C.F., Demopoulos, B., & Adelman, R.D. (2010, Feb). Combining the creative arts and the house call to teach medical students about chronic illness care. *Journal of the American Geriatrics Society, 58*(2), 346–351. http://dx.doi.org/10.1111/j.1532-5415.2009.02686.x Medline:20374408

McIntosh, P. (2010). *Action research and reflective practice: Creative and visual methods to facilitate reflection and learning.* Abingdon: Routledge.

McNiff, S. (2008). Art-based research. In J.G. Knowles & A.L. Cole (Eds.), *Handbook of the arts in qualitative research* (pp. 29–40). Thousand Oaks, CA: Sage.

Milligan, E., & Woodley, E. (2009, Apr–Jun). Creative expressive encounters in health ethics education: teaching ethics as relational engagement. *Teaching and Learning in Medicine, 21*(2), 131–139. http://dx.doi.org/10.1080/10401330902791248 Medline:19330692

Nouwen, H.J.M. (1998). *Reaching out.* London: Fount Paperbacks.

Polanyi, M. (1967). *The tacit dimension.* New York: Anchor Books.

Rodenhauser, P., Strickland, M.A., & Gambala, C.T. (2004, Summer). Arts-related activities across U.S. medical schools: a follow-up study. *Teaching and Learning in Medicine, 16*(3), 233–239. http://dx.doi.org/10.1207/s15328015tlm1603_2 Medline:15388377

Schön, D.A. (1983). *The reflective practitioner: How professionals think in action.* New York: Basic Books.

Seeley, C. (2011). Uncharted territory: Imagining a stronger relationship between the arts and action research. *Action Research, 9*(1), 83–99. http://dx.doi.org/10.1177/1476750310397061

Shapiro, J., Coulehan, J., Wear, D., & Montello, M. (2009, Feb). Medical humanities and their discontents: definitions, critiques, and implications. *Academic Medicine, 84*(2), 192–198. http://dx.doi.org/10.1097/ACM.0b013e3181938bca Medline:19174663

Sweeney, K. (2005). Science, society, suffering and the self: A commentary on general practice for the twenty-first century. *New Zealand Family Physician, 32*, 221–224.

Thompson, T., Lamont-Robinson, C., & Younie, L. (2010). 'Compulsory creativity': Rationales, recipes, and results in the placement of mandatory creative endeavour in a medical undergraduate curriculum. *Medical Education Online* [Online]. Retrieved 09 December 2010 from http://www.med-ed-online.net/index.php/meo/article/view/5394

Weller, K. (2002, Nov). Visualising the body in art and medicine: a visual art course for medical students at King's College Hospital in 1999. *Complementary Therapies in Nursing & Midwifery, 8*(4), 211–216. http://dx.doi.org/10.1054/ctnm.2002.0644 Medline:12463611

Younie, L. (2006). A *qualitative study of the contribution medical humanities can bring to medical education MSc*. Unpublished thesis. University of Bristol.

Younie, L. (2011). A *reflexive journey through arts-based inquiry in medical education*. Unpublished doctoral thesis. University of Bristol.

Younie, L. (2013). Introducing arts-based inquiry into medical education: Exploring the creative arts in health and illness. In P. McIntosh & D. Warren (Eds.), *Creativity in the classroom: Case studies in using the arts in teaching and learning in higher education* (pp. 23–39). Bristol: Intellect Publishers.

Lifelines

Art in Action for Change in Health Care

Carole Condé and Karl Beveridge

Carole Condé and Karl Beveridge are professional artists who live and work in Toronto, Ontario. They have collaborated with various trade unions and community organizations in the production of their staged photographic work over the past 25 years. Their art has been exhibited across Canada and internationally in both the trade-union movement and art galleries and museums.

They are sometimes asked by those who have participated in their projects, "Why would you want to do art about our experience when we're not important?" This comment speaks volumes about the nature of work and community life in our society, but it also addresses how people see themselves and what the dominant culture has done to that perception. Condé and Beveridge work with unions and communities as part of a larger collective process to change those perceptions. Their working relationship is based on collaborative processes mediated through the union movement or community group.

Given the present social divisions of labour, this work attempts to bridge two audiences: working people and those in the arts. The artists feel, in their work, that it is important not only to articulate the concerns and experience of working and community life but also to stand up to the sophistication of corporate culture and take into account the complexities of cultural representation.

Working with the union movement and communities has other implications. It begins to address the division of labour between wage work and creative work by demystifying the construction of each and pointing to similar social and economic constraints. It also articulates a cultural politic around the democratization of access to cultural resources.

In 1996, Beveridge became quite ill and had to spend a lengthy period in hospital. During his stay, and the period of extended care that followed, he and Condé were witnesses to the working conditions health care workers face. What was particularly frightening for them was the fact that the hospital had shifted nurses to different floors every couple of days and, as a result, they could not form any attachments to the patient; thus, they were unable to observe Beveridge's deteriorating condition. This experience motivated several projects on the subject of health care.

Theatre of Operations: A Look at Health Care in the US

Theatre of operations: A look at health care in the US (2000) consisted of 11 portraits of health care workers in different job categories: nurses, visiting nurses, OR technicians, X-ray technicians, patient-care aides, clerical staff, housekeeping staff, food-services staff and laundry workers. Each portrait, on a staged background, was accompanied by a quotation from the worker that addressed his/her working conditions—for example, "If you cut all the nurses aids and most of the secretaries, who picks up the slack? If I'm stacking drawers and running to the pharmacy who's watching the patient?" Portraits also featured statements about health care in the United States—for example, "44 million people in the U.S. have no health insurance."

The portrait/scenes were interspliced with five panels carrying a historical image and quotation on care from Native, Afro-American, Asian, Arabic and European sources. Each also has a title and an image-credit panel.

The artists met with representatives from the major health care unions in Buffalo and members of the Buffalo health care coalition to determine the general direction of the project. They then visited various worksites and met with the people working there. Health care workers were chosen by the artists and unions to represent different job categories and cultures. These workers had their portraits taken and were interviewed about their jobs and the general state of health care. Based on the various discussions and interviews, the artists developed a series of staged images about the issues and concerns raised by the workers and their unions.

It should be noted that the issue of a Canadian publicly funded care system and the US private system came up many times. The majority of workers and their unions support a public system and were disappointed to learn that the Canadian health care system was moving in the direction of the US model. Part of the motivation behind this work was to produce a statement about the US health care system, from the point of view of those who work in it, for a Canadian audience. The workers represented in the work are members of the Communications Workers of America (CWA) Locals 1168, 1133 and 1122; the Service Employees International Union (SEIU) Local 1199 Upstate; and the New York State Nurses Association (NYSNA).

"Without insurance,people are cared for differently. Not in a cruel sense, but they're treated with a different attitude. It's a business now. The poor patient suffers and the poor worker suffers."
Jo Anne Sciera, X-Ray Technologist, SEIU 1199Upstate
44 MILLION PEOPLE IN THE U.S. HAVE NO HEALTH INSURANCE

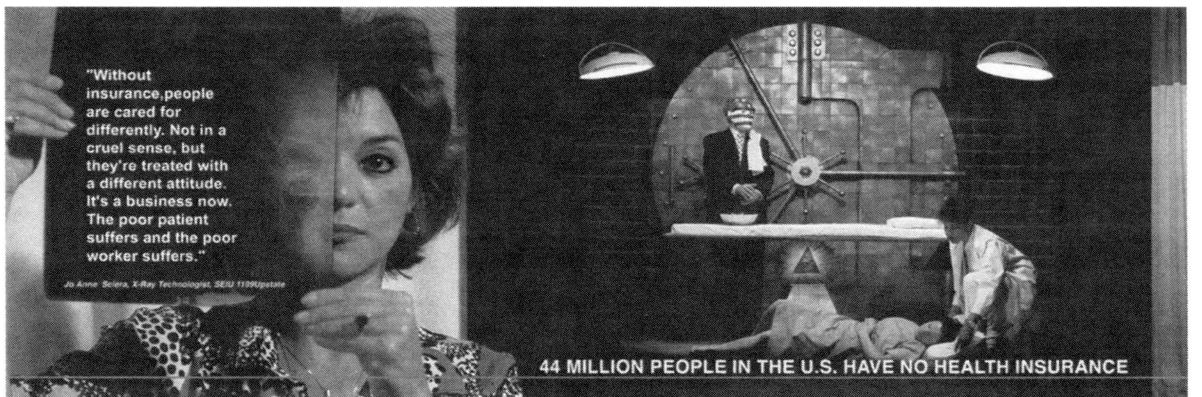

Figure L.3 Jo Anne Sciera, X-ray technologist; photo by Carol Condé and Karl Beveridge

HMO'S CONSUME UP TO 25% OF HEALTH PREMIUMS IN ADMINISTRATION
"They've doubled the paperwork and we're struggling with regulations and forms for the HMO's. And the patients want to know why this or that isn't covered and then, how they're going to pay for it."
Madaleine H. Gaume, Medical Biller, CWA 1133

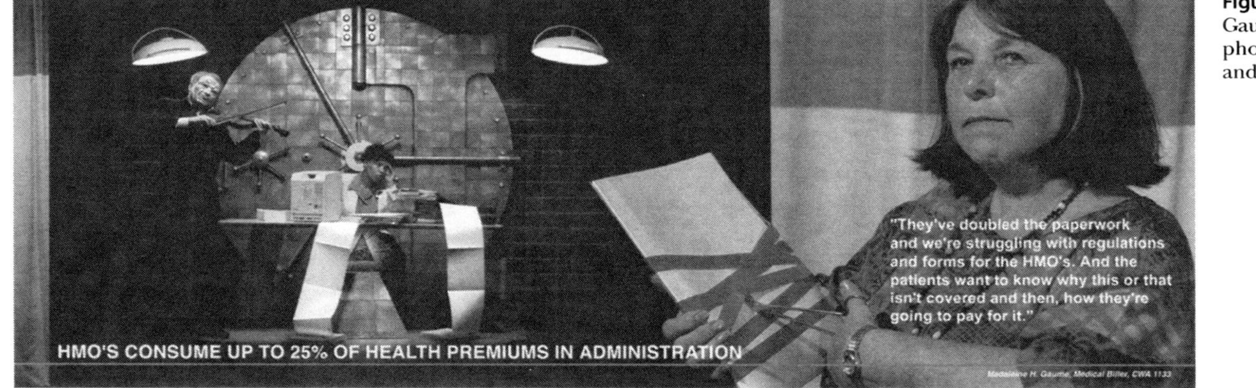

Figure L.4 Madaleine H. Gaume, medical biller; photo by Carol Condé and Karl Beveridge

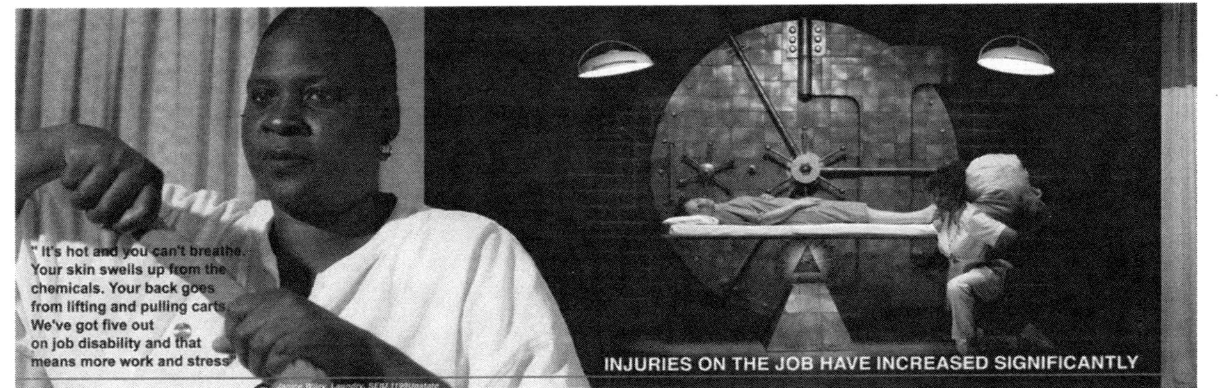

Figure L.5 Janice Wiley, laundry staff; photo by Carol Condé and Karl Beveridge

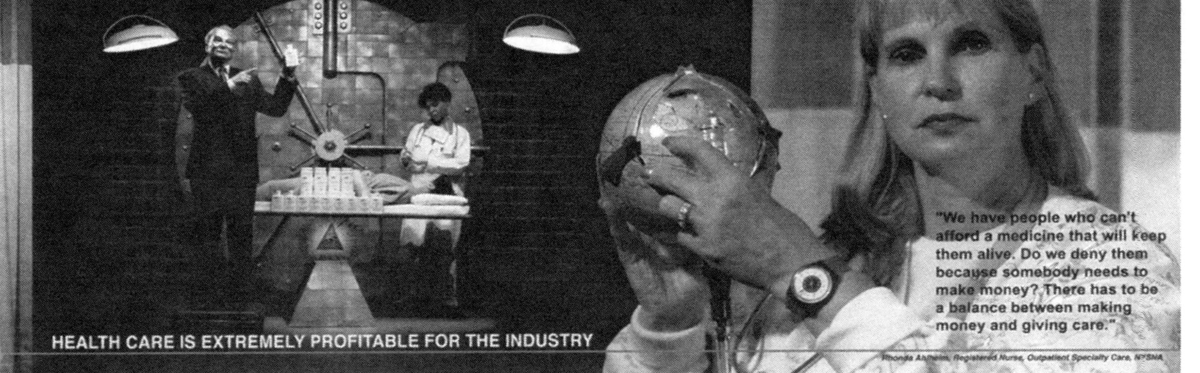

Figure L.6 Rhonda Ahlheim, RN, outpatient specialty care; photo by Carol Condé and Karl Beveridge

Ill Wind

Another health-related arts project, *Ill wind* (2001), was produced in two stages. The first stage involved a series of workshops with health care workers in Ontario, using techniques from forum theatre with the assistance of actor and director Aida Jordao. Workshops were held in Kingston (kitchen staff), Guelph (home-care workers), Hamilton (maintenance and clerical staff) and two separate workshops in Oshawa (clerical staff and nursing assistants).

Through a set of theatrical exercises the workers visualized both the work they do and their concerns about their jobs. From the image ideas gathered at the workshops, a series of five photographic concepts—one for each workshop—was developed. These concepts were then discussed and finalized with the workers. The underlying theme, expressed in different ways, was their frustration and anger over not being able to provide the care their patients needed and the stress they experience from the rising demands of the job.

The second stage involved the photographing of the final images. Two members from each of the workshops were invited to act as themselves in the images, along with actors who played the patients and management. The set was a seamless backdrop, tinted "institutional" green, with minimal props. These choices allow the viewer to focus on the workers, as well as referencing a corporate hospital environment.

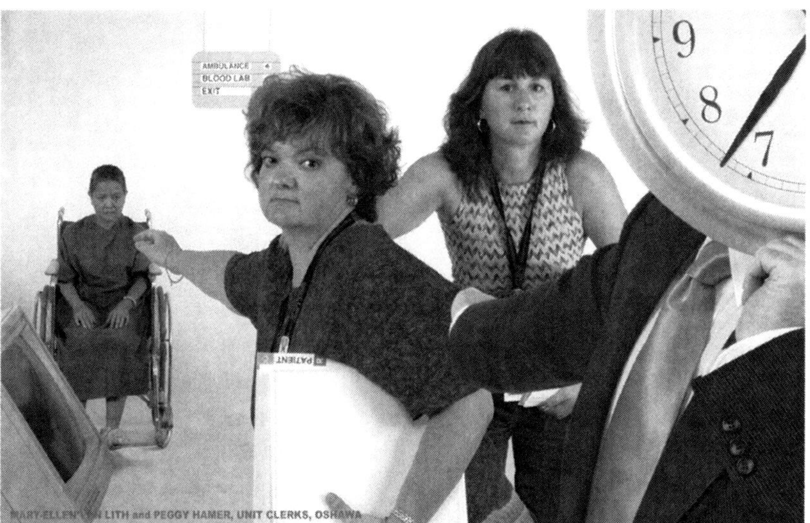

Figure L.7 Mary-Ellen Van Lith and Peggy Hamer, unit clerks; photo by Carol Condé and Karl Beveridge

The title image for *Ill wind* is a documentary of the participants in a visual workshop held in Kingston. The image *Mary-Ellen and Peggy, Oshawa* points to the stress of being caught between the demands to be more efficient and the time needed to care for a patient.

Maria and Bonnie, Guelph expresses the frustration of a worker getting an increased workload when another is laid off. *Louis and Jill, Kingston* illustrates the deskilling of kitchen staff and the loss of nutritional value when frozen meals are brought in. *Barbara and Lori, Oshawa* points to workers' need to take care of one another when under stress. *Elta and Joanne, Hamilton* demonstrates that workers are on the front lines in the fight to stop the privatization of health services in Canada.

In this project, Condé and Beveridge concentrated on collaborating with various types of workers and support staff in health care, rather than with doctors and administrators. In part, this choice reflects that they wanted to show the work of those who are often invisible in the health care system but who take great pride in their many contributions.

Both of the above projects have been used extensively by the unions involved and have been shown in various public settings. The Buffalo piece, *Theatre of operations*, was initially displayed as advertising cards around the interior and on the outside of city buses as well as back-light displays in the subway system. *Ill wind* was displayed on the Edmonton LRT transit system and was included in a mobile display (on a bus) by the union. Both works have been used extensively at union conferences and conventions as well as on placards in demonstrations in support of Medicare. In addition, the works have been included in gallery and museum exhibitions across Canada and internationally.

14

From Human Destructiveness to Creativity

Bandy X. Lee, MD

When art and education become the solid basis of a society, humanity and intelligence develop in its constituents, and this naturally restores them to health.

—*Bandy X. Lee*

Violence and destructiveness seem a ubiquitous human condition, with multitudinous harmful consequences to health. Addressing the root causes of human violence has the effect of preventing many human pathologies, leading to an improvement of population health, safety, access and distribution of medical and mental health care. Yet human violence remains an orphan topic to the medical fields, seldom given serious study. As the World Health Organization has noted that health is not merely the absence of disease, so effective violence prevention must inevitably allow human flourishing and creativity. This article underscores the importance of giving a place to the study of violence in medical education.

Claims that human violence rates have declined have recently become very popular (Pinker 2011; Eisner 2003). However, assigning simple, fixed notions to violence is problematic in itself, as it ignores the ever-changing nature of violence as life conditions change.[1] In 2000, the World Health Organization estimated that 1.6 million people lost their lives to violence, and this number has scarcely changed over the last decade despite some shifts in types of violence. Few would consider this outcome acceptable, given the knowledge we now have that many forms of violence are largely preventable. For prevention efforts to be effective, however, violence needs to be seen for the complex, changeable human phenomenon that it is, and we must give it the complex, contextual consideration it is due. Human violence is an essential topic for human pathology at a time when we are recognizing that human safety, population health and human rights are closely interrelated (for instance, as medical technologies develop, whether or not an individual will survive and thrive becomes more a matter of access to care than of safety from harm). Students of creativity often have an intuitive understanding of the causal relationship between social injustice and individual violence, and between individual creativity and social healing.[2] We can no longer leave out the study of violence prevention in medical education, for its centrality to societal and individual mental and physical health, and by extension, the study of creativity. In spring 2013, Yale College offered its first comprehensive course on violence as a part of the Global Health curriculum, covering everything from the biology, psychology and sociology of violence to the perspectives of anthropology, political science, public health, creativity studies, environment and nonviolence on the topic.

Whether the trend of human violence is decreasing or increasing, few will argue that violence levels are unacceptably high and remain a major concern, about which we have insufficient knowledge and even less understanding. Only recently the United States, so ridden with school violence and individual-driven massacres, was shocked once again with the mass murder, in a quiet Connecticut town, of innocents barely seven years old. Soon thereafter, Oscar Pistorius, an Olympic hero from South Africa, fatally shot his girlfriend, whom he claimed to love. And at the time of this writing, the suspects from a bombing at the Boston Marathon had been captured or killed. It is unsurprising that Sigmund Freud wrote, in *Civilization and its discontents* (1930), "Men are not gentle friendly creatures wishing for love ... A powerful measure for aggression has to be reckoned as part of their instinctive endowment ... *Homo homini lupus*" (p. 86). Freud held this view until his death.

Students of human creativity do not hold such a dim view. We have seen enough of human resilience, generativity, productivity and *élan vital*—to borrow Henri Bergson's phrase—to know a different kind of human potential. The problem, rather, is that we have attempted to confront violence in the past with denial and resignation, if not further violence. If we thought creatively—that is, interpersonally, diplomatically, politically, socially and culturally—violence as a "solution"—whether the source be the individual or the state—should not be necessary. An in-depth observation of the human psyche reveals that violent impulses are creative impulses gone awry, that any violent criminal would much rather create if he/she thought him/herself capable. Those who have worked closely with violent offenders make the observation again and again that violence is a result of *desperation* (offenders' prideful claims notwithstanding) and that if one truly believed one could be productive, there is no doubt which one would choose. Our creative impulse is so fundamental, so critical, as a culmination of that natural impetus in any living being, that allowing for its constructive expression would probably pull us out of more problems than we could ever imagine through mere confrontation.

The science of violence studies confirms this. Since United States Surgeon General Dr. C. Everett Koop first creatively led the health sector into the field of violence prevention, many important institutions have advocated that we approach violence as a problem in public health: the Centers for Disease Control and Prevention (CDC) of the US Public Health Service, the Institute of Medicine (IOM) of the National Academy of Sciences and the World Health Organization (WHO), among others. The investigation into violence shifted away from criminology, law and politics to public health, preventive medicine and mental health. In contrast to *retribution* of individuals after the fact, *restoration* at all levels, and positive reinforcement through community programs, mentorship, parenting classes and even improvements in prenatal care, have scientifically proven to be more effective in helping populations lead productive lives. We are beginning to see throughout the world what can happen when cultures encourage and allow individuals to participate in building and in creation through an "upstream" emphasis on prevention rather than a "downstream" approach to reacting when problems have grown into an overwhelming cascade. When art and education become the solid basis of a society, humanity and intelligence ripen in its constituents, and this development naturally restores the population to health.

Archaeological evidence supports this approach. In ancient China, apart from hereditary power, scholar officials determined the affairs of the state. These officials were in fact artists, theoretically from any background or social status, who won competitions in poetry, calligraphy and painting. Of course, learned philosophy came through in their artwork, but the purpose was to select the greatest humanists, who were assumed to have the greatest wisdom and therefore an ability to make important governing decisions. This is the kind of civilization that has become legend, one that western Europe approached during the Renaissance but has never yet fully realized.

Similarly, in ancient Africa, political systems often consisted of circles of tribal members, divided by age and gender, that would hold repeated discussions until a problem reached resolution. Other than the chief, political appointments were rare and arose primarily out of necessity. This system maintained order in a widespread, decentralized way, kept solutions at a very human (and humanistic) level and probably prevented any one individual or entity from taking over, as has occurred post-Western influence.

Evidence supports the finding that violence prevention begins with reducing inequality and injustice—in other words, with good governance. However, our current systems require such specialized knowledge to manoeuvre—all technicalities and little wisdom—that it seems the greater this knowledge, the less room there may be for a true understanding of human affairs, not to mention human solutions. A result is that rampant immorality and injustice are permitted to reign without regard to human and social casualty—the kind that any scholar official or tribal member would have long recognized as antithetical to the purpose of government. Instead, our system allows us to deny almost any problem, some of terrifying proportions: global climate change, destruction of the planet, erosion of democracy, depletion of social safety nets, plunder of the poor and illegal wars, to name just a few. We are told that the source of our problems is complex and mysterious and the solutions are beyond the reach of the average citizen. However, the participation and flourishing of the average citizen is perhaps the best indicator of a society's health.

The 17th-century philosopher Baruch Spinoza remarked in his *Theoretical–political treatise* that "Peace is not an absence of war, it is a virtue, a state of mind, a disposition for benevolence, confidence, justice." This state of mind also gives rise to creativity and allows the trend to reverse direction from the source. This perspective echoes the WHO's (1946) definition of health as "a state of complete ... well-being and not merely the absence of disease"; indeed, individuals of greater levels of mental health are more inclined to creative expression, whatever their field of choice may be. And these individuals are the source of an ethos capable of creating healthier conditions for society.

If Plato called for philosophers to become rulers for global decision-making to carry thoughtfulness, we might call upon practitioners of creativity for ethical bearing. While education empowers populations by alerting them to ways in which oppression can occur, the arts do so by centring the heart such that one will refuse to accept injustice or untruth (the role of aesthetics in ethics is not new: see Scarry, 1999). In other words, what education achieves cognitively, art does emotionally—and with most problems facing us now originating in humans, we see that we are in great need of collective emotional healing. In this context, it does not help that we marginalize artists from "Bohemia" to misery—a distant cry from the position of scholar official—for the suffering of artists often foreshadows the suffering of a whole civilization.

Thus, in developing a proper perspective for global ethics, those in the creative fields may have a crucial role to play. Few professions take on the ultimate of human expression and are sensitive to any curtailing of human thriving (Henry James, for instance, suffered with a prescience of the Second World War while everyone was rejoicing at the end of the First and politicians were emitting sighs of relief). Their sensitivity can become a guide for ethical global governance, which is the starting point of any serious attempt at preventing violence on a major scale. A humanistic approach characteristic of the arts might lead to the recognition of principles over rules, like the African governing circles that brought no concrete formula other than to answer a specific question. Amid changing conditions, keeping with original purpose can allow us not to lose sight of the basic principles that every healthy society seeks (and that keep societies healthy): harmony, equity, justice and peace. We might then work toward true prosperity rather than a mere absence of violence or war, as we take a step toward restoring our society to a higher, healthier civilization.

NOTES

1 A serious flaw in Pinker's claim, for instance, is that he leaves out suicide, an exponentially increasing form of violence in our day that is far greater than all homicides and war deaths *combined* and that is projected to double in little more than a decade.

2 A contemporary example of an explicit connection between art and social change, through the reduction of poverty, injustice and inequality in health care, can be seen in the work of Canadian photographers Carole Condé and Karl Beveridge (see condebeveridge.ca). If we go back in time, the works of Théodore Géricault and Eugène Delacroix can be said to have incited political awareness and movements, the way Rembrandt van Rijn and Bartolomé Murillo inspired humanism a couple centuries earlier.

REFERENCES

Eisner, M. (2003). Long-term historical trends in violent crime. In M. Tonry (Ed.), *Crime and justice: A review of research* (Vol. 30, pp. 83–142). Chicago: University of Chicago Press.

Freud, S. (1930). *Civilization and its discontents.* London: Hogarth Press.
Pinker, S. (2011). *The better angels of our nature: Why violence has declined.* New York: Viking.
Scarry, E. (1999). *On beauty and being just.* Princeton, NJ: Princeton University Press.
World Health Organization. (1946). *Preamble to the Constitution of the World Health Organization.* As adopted by the International Health Conference, New York, 19–22 June.

15

Digital Stories for Teaching Ethics and Law to Health and Social Service Professionals

Louise Terry

The use of stories to share notions of self and other, right and wrong, characterizes all human societies. We grow through the stories we hear even when the hearing is uncomfortable. Worldwide, health care professionals increasingly subscribe to Schön's (1986) concept of the reflective practitioner, which built on Dewey's (1933) seminal treatise. In the United Kingdom formal, assessed reflection is now part of medical education in the belief this reflection will improve empathy. Trainee family doctors are expected to complete online learning logs where they reflect on episodes of patient care and other events (Stillman, 2012).

Sometimes the stories we tell—about ourselves, about our professional practice—are not the complete truth. Stories can be distorted through a dominant paradigm that disempowers or oppresses, as identified by Hall's (2011) research, employing digital stories within a critical-literacy framework to allow young African American women in white university-educational systems to find their own voices. Hall drew on Du Bois' "double consciousness," which holds great potential for understanding the multiple faces of the patient–family–health care professional triad of which practitioners sometimes lose sight. No one is "just" a nurse, "purely" a doctor, "simply" a patient, yet this can become an overpowering paradigm that objectifies and condemns health care practitioners and the recipients of care to be compartmentalized as "nurse," "doctor," "patient," "client," "service user." This positionality means that we enter situations within the confines of a contextual subjectivity (silo thinking) (Knight, 2011) that limits our effectiveness and often our compassion. I believe that to practice humane medicine, we need to rediscover our sense of ourselves and our patients as people of differing professions, beliefs, values and politics; differing colours and ethnicities; wives, mothers, daughters, fathers, sons; imperfect, struggling to do our best, or merely just survive, within an imperfect and often unjust world.

Visual and audio technology can help bring stories, actions, omissions, aspirations and values to life and allow a permanent record of the story to be kept for future use. Digital storytelling is a useful pedagogical tool (Terry, 2012) employing the art of narrative in combination with digital media such as images, sound and video to tell a story (Dreon, Kerper & Landis, 2011). Educationally, digital storytelling can be positioned within a contemplative pedagogy that cultivates inner awareness (Grace, 2011) and embraces case studies (as described in this chapter), reflections on personal experiences, interviews, life stories, and interactions with texts, artifacts, people and situations. One UK initiative in digital storytelling is Patient Voices, a growing archive developed through facilitated small group workshops:

> to facilitate the telling and the hearing of some of the unwritten and unspoken stories of ordinary people so that those who devise and implement strategy in health and social care, as well as the professionals and clinicians directly involved in care, may carry out their duties in a more informed and compassionate manner. (Patient Voices, n.d.)

Storytelling seems as old as oral language and is a way in which customs and values are shared across generations (Coulter, Michael & Poynor, 2007). At the University of British Columbia, a community-based research project has used digital stories to archive and understand Chinese Canadian history and experience and is creating "new ideas, new concepts, and new fields of ... study" (Cho, 2011). In Australia, animated storytelling has helped non-Aboriginal teachers understand Aboriginal values and ways of knowing (McKnight, Hoban & Nielson, 2011).

In health care education, storytelling allows meaning to be derived from chaos, helps moral development and makes accessible the themes of connection and care, allowing us to enter the worlds of real people and consider how we would "think, feel and act if faced with similar situations" (McDrury & Alterio, 2002, p. 36). For example, people with learning disabilities have provided oral histories as digital stories that reveal their everyday hardship and neglect (Manning, 2010).

Using stories drawn from practice—from real patients and clients—helps personalize the learning experience. Digital stories often describe "routine and problematic moments and meanings in individuals' lives" (Guajardo et al., 2011, p. 149), the goal being to develop better understanding of human behaviour through improved knowledge of self and others. Repper and Breeze (2007) found that involving service users helps practitioners demonstrate greater empathy and understanding. However, digital stories, film and audio can be static and one sided and may lack interactivity (D'Alessandro, Lewis & D'Alessandro, 2004), so that student learning may remain shallow even if the story is analyzed in classroom discussions. The challenge for educators is to ensure that understanding is not superficial. Tooth and Renshaw (2009) argue in favour of a "slow pedagogy" (p. 98) that allows students to spend more than a fleeting moment in authentic educational experiences to listen, receive meaning and move into a deeply reflective space. They conclude that attention is the real object of education (p. 102). We need health care practitioners who pay attention to the quality of care provided, who deliver humane medicine.

I first augmented a digital story with online discussions over a two- to three-week period between my graduate students and the spinal-injured patient whose story was told. This process responded to Dewey's four conditions that maximize learning by ensuring that the story interest the learner; that it is seen as intrinsically worthwhile by the learner; that it present a problem that awakens curiosity and a desire for more information; and that it foster development over time. The central point of the patient's story was an error in nursing records when the patient reported being unable to move his left leg. The record read "Patient cannot move left leg. Says it was normal for him" when, in fact, it was not normal. This error led to a three-day delay before doctors were alerted to the problem and had to consider spinal-decompression surgery. A digital story based on the experience was shown and discussed in class, followed by online discussions with the patient through Blackboard, the university's e-learning platform. This exploration uncovered other, unreported, concerning examples of poor nursing care. One obvious example was the photo the patient took of the curtains around his bed, which were left partly open when he was given a urinal bottle, thereby embarrassing him and robbing him of his privacy. There were several photos of the food (meat, baked beans, curry and rice, suet pudding) that presented a choking risk, identified by a spinal-injuries specialist nurse who was part of the first class to view the patient's story.

There are many ways to approach a digital story. Sheneman (2010) provides a useful table comparing Photostory 3 with Animoto and MovieMaker; I prefer Photostory 3. Numerous resource websites also exist (a useful selection is available via Edina Public Schools, n.d.). One useful overview is *Digital storytelling: A tutorial in 10 easy steps* (n.d.). Sadik (2008) provides a table showing Bernard Robin's four-stage framework to creating and integrating digital stories. The basic steps are as follows: define the topic, collect materials that might be useful and start considering the purpose of the story; select the images and audio and import them into a new project in the chosen software program; decide the purpose of the story, write the script (storyboard), record the narrative and finalize the video file; demonstrate the digital story and evaluate its effectiveness. The typical digital story, according to Walters, Green, Wang and Walters (2011), is three to five minutes long and combines images, video, music and text with the narrative spoken by the author. However, digital stories about health care often run up to 10 minutes long (Patient Voices, n.d.), which is also the time limit imposed by YouTube.

YouTube is turning everyone into home video–makers. Using YouTube, we have the potential to encourage students to explore the humanity of care with their webcams and smartphones. Ensuring students can access and use existing and emerging technologies will help them personalize their learning (Demski, 2012) in ways appropriate to their learning styles (Kolb & Kolb, 2005) and help them communicate, learn and grow (Kahn & Coburn, 1998). To support this kind of learning, educators need to be supported in developing their own abilities to use and critique these technologies.

Younger people may be "digital natives" and the way they "communicate, interact, process information and learn" has certainly changed (Dreon et al., 2011, p. 4). Allowing students to develop their creative use of technology to support their own and others' learning is the future of health care education, but the paramount principle must always remain: "First, do no harm." Students could focus on episodes of care observed, experienced or given, and the process of constructing their digital story could help them construct their own meanings from thinking about the experiences (Sadik, 2008, p. 488). Some health students might even create their own web series to distribute via Blip.tv or a similar service.

Educationally, my approach to digital storytelling is underpinned by constructivism, which acknowledges that the health care we deliver is not practiced in an ideal world; silo thinking and personal, professional, organizational and societal constraints limit our understanding and humanity. I seek to help my students understand this idea for themselves through reflective engagement with real stories and real people, interpreted through theoretical constructs (which in my specialty are related to ethics, law and professional practice), not merely personal constructs, and thereby becoming active conceptualizers who can "collaborate and reflectively co-construct new understandings" (Ukpokodu, 2008). Most important, I hope their educational experience will be transformational, shifting their perspectives so they become better, more competent and more compassionate health care practitioners.

REFERENCES

Cho, A. (2011). Bringing history to the library: University–community engagement in the academic library. *Computers in Libraries, 31*(4), 15–18.

Coulter, C., Michael, C., & Poynor, L. (2007). Storytelling as pedagogy: An unexpected outcome of narrative inquiry. *Curriculum Inquiry, 37*(2), 103–122. http://dx.doi.org/10.1111/j.1467-873X.2007.00375.x

D'Alessandro, D.M., Lewis, T.E., & D'Alessandro, M.P. (2004, Jul 19). A pediatric digital storytelling system for third year medical students: The virtual pediatric patients. *BMC Medical Education, 4*, 10. Retrieved from http://www.biomedcentral.com. http://dx.doi.org/10.1186/1472-6920-4-10 Medline:15260883

Demski, J. (2012). This time, it's personal. *Technological Horizons in Education, 39*(1), 33–36.

Dewey, J. (1933). *How we think: A restatement of the relation of reflective thinking to the educative process (Rev. ed.).* Boston: D.C. Heath.

Digital Storytelling: A tutorial in 10 easy steps. (n.d.). Retrieved from http://www.socialbrite.org/2010/07/15/digital-storytelling-a-tutorial-in-10-easy-steps/

Dreon, O., Kerper, R.M., & Landis, J. (2011). Digital storytelling: A tool for teaching and learning in the YouTube generation. *Middle School Journal, 42*(5), 4–9.

Edina Public Schools. (n.d.). *Technology resources for schools.* Retrieved from https://sites.google.com/site/edinatechresources/digital-storytelling

Grace, F. (2011). Learning as a path, not a goal: Contemplative pedagogy — its principles and practices. *Teaching Theology and Religion, 14*(2), 99–124. http://dx.doi.org/10.1111/j.1467-9647.2011.00689.x

Guajardo, M., Oliver, J.A., Roderíquez, G., Valadez, M.M., Cantú, Y., & Guajardo, F. (2011). Reframing the praxis of school leadership preparation through digital storytelling. *Journal of Research on Leadership Education, 6*(5), 145–161.

Hall, T. (2011). Designing from their own social worlds: The digital story of three African American young women. *English Teaching: Practice and Critique, 10*(1), 7–20.

Kahn, F. & Coburn, J. (1998). Clips from the heart. *Technology & Learning, 18*(9), 52–56.

Knight, S.D. (2011). Using narrative to examine positionality: Powerful pedagogy in English education. *English Teaching: Practice and Critique, 10*(2), 49–64.

Kolb, A.Y., & Kolb, D.A. (2005). Learning styles and learning spaces: Enhancing experiential learning in higher education. *Academy of Management Learning & Education, 4*(2), 193–212. http://dx.doi.org/10.5465/AMLE.2005.17268566

Manning, C. (2010). "My memory's back!" Inclusive learning disability research using ethics, oral history and digital storytelling. *British Journal of Learning Disabilities, 38*(3), 160–167. http://dx.doi.org/10.1111/j.1468-3156.2009.00567.x

McDrury, J., & Alterio, M. (2002). *Learning through storytelling in higher education: Using reflection and experience to improve learning.* London: Kegan Page.

McKnight, A., Hoban, G., & Nielson, W. (2011). Using Slowmation for animated storytelling to represent non-Aboriginal preservice teachers' awareness of "relatedness to country." *Australian Journal of Educational Technology, 27*(1), 41–54.

Patient Voices. (n.d.). From http://www.patientvoices.org.uk/

Repper, J., & Breeze, J. (2007, Mar). User and carer involvement in the training and education of health professionals: A review of the literature. *International Journal of Nursing Studies, 44*(3), 511–519. http://dx.doi.org/10.1016/j.ijnurstu.2006.05.013 Medline:16842793

Sadik, A. (2008). Digital storytelling: A meaningful technology-integrated approach for engaged student learning. *Educational Technology Research and Development, 56*(4), 487–506. http://dx.doi.org/10.1007/s11423-008-9091-8

Schön, D.A. (1986). *Educating the reflective practitioner: Toward a new design for teaching and learning in the professions.* San Francisco, CA: Jossey-Bass.

Sheneman, L. (2010). Digital storytelling: How to get the best results. *School Library Monthly, 27*(1), 40–42.

Stillman, K. (2012). A *service evaluation of the nMRCGP e-portfolio learning log as an educational tool for developing reflective practice in GP trainees.* Unpublished master's dissertation. London: London South Bank University, United Kingdom.

Terry, L.M. (2012, Feb). Service user involvement in nurse education: A report on using online discussions with a service user to augment his digital story. *Nurse Education Today, 32*(2), 161–166. http://dx.doi.org/10.1016/j.nedt.2011.06.006 Medline: 21737188

Tooth, R., & Renshaw, R. (2009). Reflections on pedagogy and place: A journey into learning for sustainability through environmental narrative and deep attentive reflection. *Australian Journal of Environmental Education, 25*, 95–104.

Ukpokodu, O.N. (2008). Teachers' reflections on pedagogies that enhance learning in an online course on teaching for equality and social justice. *Journal of Interactive Online Learning, 7*(3), 227–255.

Walters, L., Green, M., Wang, L., & Walters, T. (2011). From heads to hearts: Digital stories as reflection artefacts of teachers' international experience. *Issues in Teacher Education, 20*(2), 37–52.

Lifelines

Reaching Out with Heartfelt Art

Medical and Fine Arts Students Build Bridges to Communities

Carol Ann Courneya

"The visual arts have the power to transform space from utility to something which embodies the higher ideals of that space, to imbue them with vibrancy as opposed to the lifeless bare walls of an institution," wrote a University of British Columbia (UBC) medical student. These words formed the core mission of a unique collaborative project that brought together medical and fine arts students to co-create art for community health centres in Vancouver.

> I was attracted to the "Heartfelt Images" in the cardiac unit. I have just been discharged from the Healthy Heart Clinic for good behaviour, part of that is art therapy. I saw a thread of my journey in those images and it made me feel good.

This quotation comes from a cardiac patient at Vancouver General Hospital in reference to the display of winning submissions from an annual cardiac-art contest called "Heartfelt Images," in which medical and dental students conceptualize artistically what they learn about the heart and circulatory system (Courneya, 2009).

Admission to medical school is often tied to the applicant's well roundedness: academic prowess, social accountability, empathy, artistic and athletic talents. Yet once students are accepted to the program, medical school is—both by reputation and in fact—a time for students to buckle down, burn the midnight oil, hit the books. Recent studies, however, make it abundantly clear that building in elective or curricular opportunities for medical students to engage with art and humanities fosters increased empathy, as well as enhanced communication and observational skills (Bardes, Gillers & Herman, 2001; Naghshineh, Hafler, Miller et. al, 2008; Taylor, 1981; Shapiro, Nguyen, Mourra, Ross, Thai & Leonard, 2006).

Building Bridges

The Doctor, Patient and Society (Self-Directed) Project at UBC was conceived of as an opportunity to bring arts and medical students together with a common aim: to co-create art that would hang in community health centres around the city of Vancouver. The objectives were to foster creativity (art-making) and enhanced communication skills (student to student and students to community stakeholders). Students enrolled in UBC's Doctor, Patient and Society course partnered with students enrolled in a fourth-year studio course at UBC Faculty of Arts as well as students at Emily Carr University of Art and Design. After an initial "meet and greet," the medical/art student pairs selected a community health centre, engaged in an iterative art-planning process and co-created and installed the art in the centres. In two of the projects the students worked with residents of the centres in creating their own art.

Throughout the project the medical students kept reflective journals and met periodically to update their project tutor regarding the barriers in and successes of the project. Achieving success in this project was tied largely to collaborative and communication skills. Art students and medical students needed to establish a common dialogue, acknowledging and working with the different skill sets they brought to the table. In a pre-course questionnaire one medical student wrote, "I'm nervous about collaborating. What if the [art] student isn't overly flexible? What if I don't like what they're doing? What if I may have specific ideas that they don't like?" Layered on this peer-to-peer communication was the necessity for the pairs to engage in a meaningful way with the administrators of the community health centres. In some cases that meant one-on-one discussions with centre directors. In larger centres it meant submitting formal written proposals to art committees. In all cases it required sometimes-frustrating negotiation to satisfy both the artistic vision of the student pairs and the fit with the mission and goals of the centres. One student said,

> the most valuable part as well as the most frustrating part of the project, was dealing with the bureaucratic red tape in trying to decide with a centre what they want, what will be created, and where it will go. I think it was good in the sense that it helps you understand how convoluted the hierarchy can get in health care/community centres and hospitals.

The students were the primary managers of their artwork and had to ensure that deliverables were met at the end of each term. The students also aspired to advocate for improved patient experiences within community health centres by making them more inviting and comforting. One student remarked,

> I had a chance to experience and truly appreciate how art can be of help and hope for numerous hurt and distressed people. It will continue to evolve, as there will be more clients' arts and more memories of deceased clients added to the albums and to the healing room. We hope that it will continue to initiate hope and healing in many people in the future.

The students hoped patients would be able to relate to the artwork and as a result generate conversations between patients and health care workers.

Ultimately, anxieties were overcome, barriers were broken down and stereotypes (med student versus art student, students versus administrators) were explored and set aside. In the end more than 25 pieces of art were co-created. Far beyond the art produced or the grades achieved, the students built new bridges to learning, and centre residents saw the students and themselves as creative and talented human beings (Courneya, 2013).

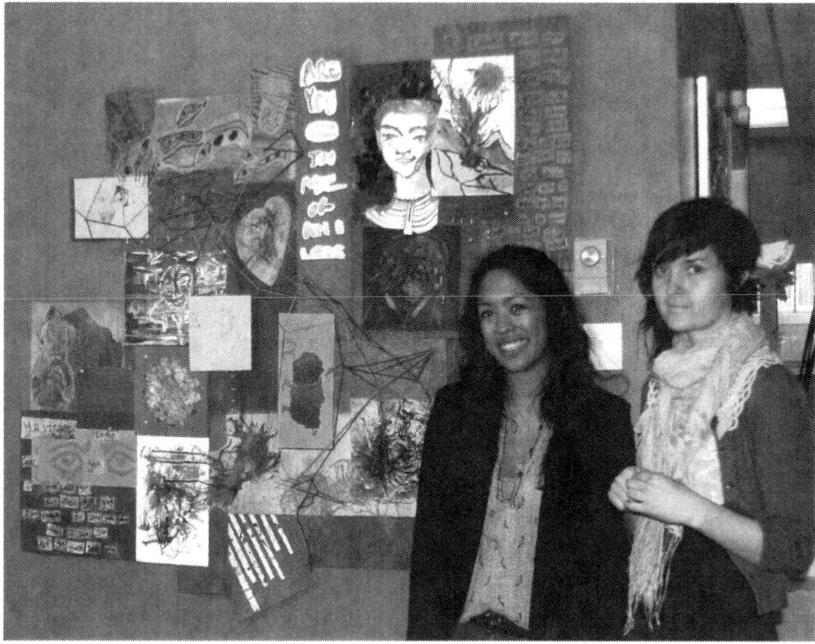

Figure L.8 Samantha Wong (UBC Medicine) and Nicole Westman (Emily Carr University of Art and Design) in front of their collage of original art created by residents of First United Mission (Vancouver East Side)

Heartfelt Images

Heartfelt Images is another project at UBC, an annual cardiac art contest that provides a platform for medical/dental students to embrace and be celebrated for their artistic and creative talents (Courneya, 2009). The five-week contest runs in conjunction with the cardiac block during first year. It produces about 150 submissions annually from a class of 280. A unique aspect of this contest is that the art is judged as much for its artistic qualities (composition, colour, innovation, skill) as for its illustration of cardiac scientific concepts. Examples from past contest winners have included *Heart murmur* (the sound heard with a stethoscope captured artistically as playful spirits inside the heart), *Polymorphic ventricular tachycardia* (a very fast and irregular heart rate seen by the student's artistic eye as boats at a marina) and *Spirit of the heart* (four animals that form an anatomically perfect heart).

In 2012 I was invited to print, frame and hang winning images from the past 13 years of the Heartfelt Images contest. These images now

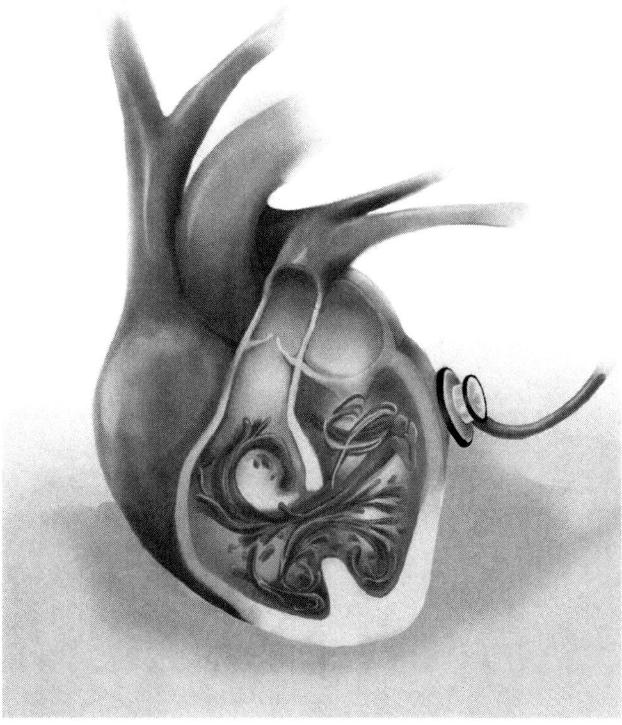

Figure L.9 *Heart murmur* by Julia Lin

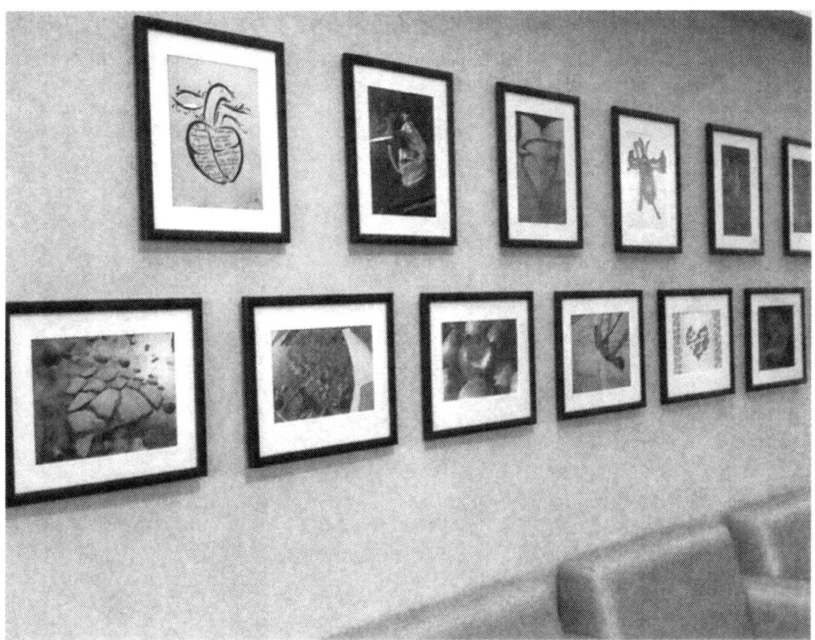

Figure L.10 Heartfelt Images hanging in the Cardiac Care Unit waiting room

grace the waiting room outside the Cardiac Care Unit in a UBC teaching hospital.

Shortly after the images were installed, an e-mail arrived from a cardiac patient for whom the cardiac art was a revelation. When asked why the art had made such an impression on him, he told a story about encountering the colder side of medicine through interactions with doctors whose bedside manner was at times lacking. He said the images made him realize that there were doctors out there who felt, as he did, that art has a role in healing, and the realization had left him profoundly "encouraged."

This patient's comment brought the art full circle: from something initially done to enhance medical students' creativity and learning to a way of connecting meaningfully with patients and their own personal healing journeys.

Art and art-making have the power to transform and enrich the lives of medical students, practitioners and patients (Courneya, 2011a, 2011b; Maruyama, 2012). Art starts a dialogue; it touches the place inside us that is most human and connects us—not as professionals or patients but as people.

NOTE

I would like to acknowledge the assistance of Dr. Sue Mills, Clinical Associate Professor, School of Populations and Public Health, University of British Columbia; Ms. Sandra Semchuck, Associate Professor, Faculty of Visual Art and Material Practice, Emily Carr University of Art and Design; and Mr. Barrie Jones, Lecturer, Visual Art Faculty, University of British Columbia.

REFERENCES

Bardes, C.L., Gillers, D., & Herman, A.E. (2001, Dec). Learning to look: Developing clinical observational skills at an art museum. *Medical Education, 35*(12), 1157–1161. http://dx.doi.org/10.1046/j.1365-2923.2001.01088.x Medline:11895244

Courneya, C.A. (2009). Heartfelt images. *University of Alberta Health Sciences Journal, 5*(1), 13–17.

Courneya, C.A. (2011a, Nov). On teaching confidence and creativity. *Medical Education, 45*(11), 1070–1071. http://dx.doi.org/10.1111/j.1365-2923.2011.04130.x Medline:21988622

Courneya, C.A. (2011b). White coat warm art: A celebration of health sciences creativity from coast to coast. *Ars Medici, 8*, 81–85.

Courneya, C.A. (2013). White coat, warm art. In D.J. Salter (Ed.), *Cases on Quality Teaching Practices in Higher Education* (pp. 106–118). Hershey, PA: IGI Global. http://dx.doi.org/10.4018/978-1-4666-3661-3.ch007

Maruyama, M. (2012, Sep 4). Medical doodles: 30 minutes well spent. Interview by Carol Ann Courneya. *Canadian Medical Association Journal, 184*(12), 1395–1396. http://dx.doi.org/10.1503/cmaj.111453 Medline:23110277

Naghshineh, S., Hafler, J.P., Miller, A.R., et al. (2008, Jul). Formal art observation training improves medical students' visual diagnostic skills. *Journal of General Internal Medicine, 23*(7), 991–997. http://dx.doi.org/10.1007/s11606-008-0667-0 Medline:18612730

Shapiro, J., Nguyen, V., Mourra, S., Ross, M., Thai, T., & Leonard, R. (2006). The use of creative projects in a gross anatomy class. *Journal for Learning through the Arts, 2*(1). http://www.escholarship.org/uc/item/3mj728bn

Taylor, J. (1981). *Learning to look: A handbook for the visual arts.* Chicago: University of Chicago Press.

Contributors

Rachael Allen is a visual artist living and working in Newcastle upon Tyne, UK. On achieving a first-class honours degree in fine art, Rachael established an expertise in drawing and miniature model making. She exhibits regularly nationwide and internationally and achieves artwork sales, commissions and residencies. Currently artist in residence at three university anatomy labs in northeast England (Newcastle, Northumbria and Durham), she is orchestrating various projects exploring the role of visual art in anatomy and medical pedagogy while situating her practice within the medical humanities nationwide. She is also involved in arts-related community work and public-engagement projects as a director and senior artist at the contemporary participatory arts enterprise Dot to Dot Active Arts.

Associate Professor **Mina Borromeo** is a specialist in Special Needs Dentistry (SND) and Convener of SND at the Melbourne Dental School, University of Melbourne. She completed her undergraduate training at the Melbourne Dental School in 1991. She also holds a PhD in muscle physiology from Monash University and a master's of science in pain medicine from Sydney University, and is a Fellow in the Faculty of Pain Medicine, Australian and New Zealand College of Anaesthetists and the Royal Australian College of Dental Surgeons (Special Needs Dentistry). Mina has worked and researched extensively in the field of dentistry and is passionate about those with special needs. She has received two NHMRC major research grants, numerous ADRF grants and a major grant from Novartis pharmaceuticals. She was the recipient of the

Andrew Vern Barnett prize in SND and has twice been awarded the New Zealand Hospital Dentists Conference prize for best presentation. She is currently president of the Australian and New Zealand Academy of Special Needs Dentistry and has been past president of the Australian Academy of Orofacial Pain.

Craig Chen, MD, is an anesthesiology resident at Stanford University Medical Center. He graduated from Stanford University with a BA in philosophy and with a BS in biological sciences and a minor in creative writing. He completed his medical degree at the University of California, San Francisco. He writes poetry and creative nonfiction for his medical blog, *Asclepion*. He received a Healing Arts Poetry Scholarship to attend the 2009 Napa Valley Writers' Conference, where he worked with David St. John.

Neville Chiavaroli, BAppSc, BA (Hons), MPhil, MEd, is a senior lecturer in medical education in the Melbourne Medical School at the University of Melbourne. Originally trained as a physiotherapist, he subsequently moved into educational development and research. Neville worked for several years at the Australian Council for Educational Research, where he was involved in developing resources and assessments in the Humanities and Social Sciences for school and university contexts, as well as admissions tests for medicine and other health professions. He joined the Melbourne Medical School in 2006 and is chiefly involved in curriculum and assessment design and review of the MD course. His main interests are in assessment and validity, medical admissions and the role of the humanities in health professional education.

Amy Clements-Cortés, PhD, MusM, MTA, MT-BC, FAMI, is currently the president of the Canadian Association for Music Therapy; an academic advisor and sessional instructor of music therapy, University of Windsor; contract academic staff and clinical supervisor, Wilfrid Laurier University; and Senior Music Therapist/Practice Advisor at Baycrest Centre, Toronto. Dr. Clements-Cortés began her career as a music therapist, performer and vocal teacher and obtained her master's and doctoral degrees from the University of Toronto. She has worked extensively in geriatrics, adult mental health, complex continuing care, palliative care and oncology, and has experience with survivors of the Holocaust. Her work has been presented around the world and published in peer-reviewed journals. Dr. Clements-Cortés has produced several recordings, among them *Soothing Relaxation Journeys* and *Episodes of Relationship Completion*. She is Clinical Commissioner for the World Federation of Music Therapy and chairperson and member of the board of directors for the Room 217 Foundation. Her music studio Notes By Amy was founded in 1995. Visit www.notesbyamy.com for more details.

Canadian artists **Carole Condé** and **Karl Beveridge** moved to New York City in 1969 and soon were at the centre of the burgeoning conceptual art movement. In 1975, they joined the art and language journal *The Fox* (with Joseph Kosuth and Ian Burn) and picketed the Museum of Modern Art to protest its lack of inclusion of women artists, while critiquing the apolitical minimalism of Donald Judd. This ferment culminated in a major museum show, *It's Still Privileged Art*, at the Art Gallery of Ontario in 1976, just before the artists' return to Toronto in 1977. By the late 1970s, Condé and Beveridge drew a focus on various issues that were urgent within the trade union movement. Their method of working dialogically with their subjects was invented for the landmark 1981 project *Standing Up* and has been refined in numerous subsequent collaborations. In the past three decades, more than 50 solo exhibitions of Condé and Beveridge's work have been presented at major museums and art spaces on four continents, including the Institute of Contemporary Art (London, UK), Museum Folkswang (Germany), George Meany Centre (Washington), Dazibao Gallery (Montreal), Centro Cultural Recoleta (Buenos Aires), Art Gallery of Edmonton and the Australian Centre for Photography (Sydney). Equally, and congruent with the artists' commitment to accessibility, their work has been displayed in a host of non-art and public settings, such as union halls, bus shelters and bookworks, and on billboards. The artists continue to work and live in Toronto. See their website condebeveridge.ca.

Christopher Cooper, MSc, PhD Candidate, Psychology, completed his BSc in psychology at the University of Saskatchewan, where he now lectures on topics in psychology for undergraduate courses. He continued his education for a MSc in personality and a PhD in health psychology in Tallinn, Estonia, where he also studied in a private school for Jungian analytical psychology.

Carol Ann Courneya is Associate Professor in the Faculty of Medicine at the University of British Columbia. She holds a UBC Killam Teaching Award and a 3M National Teaching Fellowship. Her textbook *Cardiovascular Physiology* is used as a standard for teaching clinically relevant cardiovascular physiology. She founded (2001) and has directed the Heartfelt Images project for more than a decade. In addition, Dr. Courneya founded and co-directs a national art exhibit called *White Coat Warm Art* that showcases art created by health sciences students, residents and faculty from across Canada. Drs. Courneya and Pamela Brett-McLean (founding director) co-direct the Arts, Humanities, Social Sciences in Medicine Special Interest Group for the Canadian Association of Medical Education (CAME). Dr. Courneya has had a decade-long commitment to the development and implementation of the Patan Academy of Health Sciences (PAHS) in Kathmandu, Nepal, where she currently co-directs the cardiovascular block for first-year PAHS medical students. This is the second year for their Cardio Art Contest, called Meru Mutu Mero Kala (My Heart My Art). For more details, see www.heartfelt.med.ubc.ca.

Virginia S. Cowen, PhD, is the Director of Education at the Institute for Complementary and Alternative Medicine, where she oversees the MSHS in

Integrative Health and Wellness. She previously held academic appointments teaching massage therapy and exercise science. Dr. Cowen received her PhD from Arizona State University, her MA from Columbia University and her BS from the Indiana University School of Music. She is an exercise physiologist, massage therapist, yoga teacher and fitness instructor. She holds certifications from the NCBTMB, Pilates Method Alliance, National Strength and Conditioning Association, American College of Sports Medicine and American Council on Exercise, and is a registered yoga teacher. Dr. Cowen regularly presents at conferences and has conducted original research on massage, yoga, physical activity and health behaviour.

Jane Gair is a tutor for the Problem-Based Learning and Doctor, Patient and Society courses at the Island Medical Program (IMP), with a particular interest in teaching students about patient empathy. Dr. Gair is also the faculty development coordinator for the IMP.

Heather Gaunt has a background in music, fine arts, museum studies and history. She completed her bachelor of music (1990), bachelor of arts (Hons) (1991) and postgraduate diploma of art curatorial studies (1992) at the University of Melbourne, and her PhD in history at the University of Tasmania (2010). Heather has worked in museums since the early 1990s in curatorial and collections management roles, in the fields of international prints and drawings, Australian art and indigenous cultures. She currently holds the position of Curator of Academic Programs (Research) at the Ian Potter Museum of Art, University of Melbourne. Heather has received several scholarships and awards, including the Harold Wright Scholarship to study in the Prints and Drawings Department at the British Museum, London (1994), a research fellowship to study Australian book collections at the State Library of Tasmania (2005), the Australian Historical Association/CAL Postgraduate History Essay Prize (2008) and, most recently, the Bronwyn Jane Adams Memorial Award (University of Melbourne) (2012) to undertake international research on using art collections to teach observation skills in the field of health education. Her research interests are Australian cultural history, the history of the book, library and museum history, and education in art-museum contexts.

Julie Good, MD, DABMA, is Clinical Associate Professor of Pediatric Pain and Symptom Management at Stanford University and Director of the Inpatient Pain Service at Lucile Packard Children's Hospital at Stanford. Since 2005, the Hart Foundation has supported Dr. Good's work in the Palliative Care Program. She is Packard's first board-certified physician in Hospice and Palliative Medicine, and she directs both palliative care and pain-management education. Originally from Minnesota, she earned a bachelor of science, magna cum laude, in child development and then completed her MD studies at the University of Minnesota. Following pediatric residency, fellowship training in pediatric pain management and medical acupuncture at Stanford University, she joined the clinical faculty in 2000. As a pediatrician, poet and mother of three, Julie supports compassionate care and reflective practice in those who care for children living with life-threatening illness.

Natalya Hasan, MD, is a resident in anesthesiology at Stanford University Medical Center. Born and raised in New Jersey, she received a bachelor of arts in religious studies from Columbia University. She later conducted social work research focused on drug-and-alcohol interventions for high-risk adolescents and teens. She graduated from New York University School of Medicine in 2009. After completing an internal medicine internship at Highland Hospital, she began her residency at Stanford University.

Diane Kaufman, MD, is the founder and guiding leader of Creative Arts Healthcare—The University Hospital. A Phi Beta Kappa of Mount Holyoke College, she attended Downstate Medical Center for her medical degree followed by full training in pediatrics and psychiatry at NYU/Bellevue Hospital. She is Assistant Professor of Psychiatry and Pediatrics, a child psychiatrist and the Senior Psychiatrist at the University of Medicine and Dentistry of New Jersey—New Jersey Medical School—University Behavioral HealthCare in Newark. Dr. Kaufman is a Master Clinician at University Behavioral Healthcare and was an honoured recipient of the Healthcare Foundation of New Jersey's Leonard Tow Humanism in Medicine Award (2000) and the Lester Z. Lieberman Humanism in Healthcare Award (2011). She is the UMDNJ liaison to the New Jersey Council for the Humanities' Literature and Medicine Program. A published poet and expressive-arts educational facilitator with expertise in therapeutic uses of poetry, she is the author of *Cracking Up and Back Again: Transformation Through Poetry* and *Bird That Wants To Fly*, a children's story about healing from trauma. Dr. Kaufman presents nationally and internationally on arts and healing.

Peter Kirk is a palliative care physician who researches communication in palliative care. Dr. Kirk is currently Clinical Professor with the Department of Family Practice at the University of British Columbia.

Bandy X. Lee, MD, MDiv, is a violence studies specialist. She trained as a psychiatrist at Yale and Harvard universities and focused on public-sector work as chief resident; she was active in anthropological research in East Africa as a fellow of the National Institute of Mental Health. In addition, she worked in several maximum-security prisons throughout the United States, consulted with governments in Ireland and France and helped to set up violence prevention programs both in the US and abroad. She is currently Assistant Clinical Professor, Law and Psychiatry Division, Yale University, and teaches students representing prisoners and asylum seekers through Yale Law School. She also served as Director of Research for the Center for the Study of Violence, as consultant to the World Health Organization and as speaker to the World Economic Forum. Her interests are in public health approaches and trans-disciplinary research/discourse, and she organizes an annual colloquium series called *Making Sense* to bring together the arts, the sciences and the practical disciplines.

Catherine L. Mah, MD, FRCPC, PhD, is a scientist at the Centre for Addiction and Mental Health, Head of the Food Policy Research Initiative at the Ontario Tobacco Research Unit and Assistant Professor in the Division of Public Health Policy at the Dalla Lana School of Public Health, University of Toronto. As a practitioner, researcher and teacher, Dr. Mah is interested in how values shape public-health policy within a reflexive health practice context. Dr. Mah is currently leading several CIHR-funded projects that examine contemporary food systems and food-policy debates, is engaged in research partnerships with Toronto Public Health and the Toronto Food Strategy and is a member of the Toronto Food Policy Council.

M. Michiko Maruyama is currently a medical student at the University of British Columbia Northern Medical Program. Prior to starting medical school, Michiko completed an industrial design degree at the University of Alberta. In addition to studying medicine, she is continuing to explore art and design. For more information, see www.artoflearning.ca.

Phyllis McGee is a Research Associate with the University of Victoria's Centre on Aging. Dr. McGee is also Project Site Coordinator for the Canadian Driving Research Initiative for Vehicular Safety in the Elderly (Candrive).

Maura McIntyre, EdD, is a SSHRC post-doctoral fellow at the Centre for Arts Informed Research in the Department of Adult Education, Community Development and Counselling Psychology, Ontario Institute for Studies in Education (OISE), University of Toronto. The substantive focus of her research is Alzheimer's disease, specifically the psychosocial dimensions of care and caregiving and the contexts in which lives with dementia are lived. Her current explorations of alterative research processes and forms of representations include three-dimensional installation art, photonarrative and performance.

Cheryl L. McLean, BA, MA, CAT, independent scholar and editor of the book *Creative Arts in Humane Medicine,* completed undergraduate studies in social sciences at the University of Western Ontario and a master of arts at Concordia University. She is publisher of the open-access, peer-reviewed journal *International Journal of the Creative Arts in Interdisciplinary Practice* and is also editor of the books *Creative Arts in Interdisciplinary Practice: Inquiries for Hope and Change* (2010) and *Creative Arts in Research for Community and Cultural Change* (2011), published by Detselig/Temeron Press (now Brush Education Inc.). She has taught the course Creative Responses to Death and Bereavement at the University of Western Ontario and has special interests in the creative arts in interdisciplinary research and education, arts in medicine, practitioner wellness and ethnodrama for social change. She is also an actor and trained drama therapist. Recognized as an international leader and contributor to the field of the creative arts in interdisciplinary research, McLean has been a featured keynote speaker, lecturer, performer and workshop facilitator at national conferences and events across Canada and in the United States. She was also a guest facilitator for the American Medical Student Association's Medical Humanities Scholars Program, Perceptions of Physicians in Literature and the Arts. She is currently working with social service agencies in her home community of London, Ontario, developing a play about the experiences of women inmates in prison. E-mail: CherylMcLean@ijcaip.com. More information: CherylMcLean.com.

Alim Nagji, MD, BHSc, has been an avid actor, producer and writer for several years and founded his own production company, BackRowProduction. In 2010, as a second year medical student at the University of Alberta, he conceived of and helped to pilot a six-session, theatre-based special studies module directed to first-year students, the success of which led to the inclusion of an ongoing, formal elective option in the undergraduate medical program. His passion for teaching is fuelled by his strong desire to impart enhanced communication skills to medical students, recognizing the integral role they play in anchoring the patient–physician relationship. He is currently a resident in family medicine and hopes to integrate his scholarly interest in the medical humanities and his international work experience in his future practice.

Jodi Rabinowitz, MA, RDT, is a registered drama therapist and trauma-centred clinician. She is a graduate from NYU's drama therapy program and has worked in diverse settings such as in-patient acute-care units, hospice and out-patient clinics. She is trained in trauma-focused psychotherapy and was a clinician at the Post Traumatic Stress Center in New Haven, Connecticut. She works with children, adults and families who have experienced traumatic events in their lives. In addition to clinical work, Jodi often facilitates vicarious trauma and educational workshops for clinicians and health care providers.

Aliye Runyan, MD, Education and Research Fellow, American Medical Student Association, is the founder and director, from 2008 to 2011, of the AMSA Medical Humanities Scholars program. She is a 2012 graduate of the University of Miami-Miller School of Medicine and has held national coordinator positions within the Humanistic Medicine, Wellness and Student Life, Medical Professionalism and Medical Education action committees, and was immediate past national chair of the Medical Education team. In 2010, she moved to Maryland for a year to complete a Howard Hughes Medical Institute–NIH research fellowship, studying the role of osmotic transport pathways in uterine fibroid growth. While in her AMSA fellowship year, Aliye is applying to Ob/Gyn residency programs and has interests in family planning, international maternal-fetal health and medical education.

Marilynn Schneider, BA, is Founding Director of the Jewish Service for the Developmentally Disabled (JSDD) WAE (Wellness, Arts, Enrichment) Center. Marilynn earned her BA in anthropology at Montclair State University and has worked in the field of personal development (health, healing and spirituality) since 1981. Beginning as a practitioner of Rebenfeld Synergy Method (RSM) body/mind therapy, she then became a chaplain with Joint Chaplaincy UJC MetroWest Inc., bringing her to JSDD and the community she now serves. Coming to JSDD as Judaic Coordinator and Chaplain, Marilynn assumed the position of Director of Residential Services. The WAE Center began with a 2002 pilot program to address the reality that people with disabilities have talent and desire to create fulfilling lives. In 2004, with a grant from the Healthcare Foundation of New Jersey, the doors of the WAE Center officially opened. As founder of this cutting-edge program, Marilynn has created a synergistic approach in which quality of life is foremost. That work has expanded to include people with acquired disabilities through a program using the modalities of yoga, meditation and creative writing to increase self-image and self-worth. With each endeavour, Marilynn's pursuit of health, healing and meaningful life for individuals with disabilities is daily changing lives.

Audrey Shafer, MD, is Professor of Anesthesia, Stanford University School of Medicine; staff anesthesiologist, Palo Alto Veterans Affairs Health Care System; and Director, Arts, Humanities and Medicine Program, Stanford Center for Biomedical Ethics. Born in Philadelphia, she studied at Harvard, Stanford and the University of Pennsylvania for biochemistry, medicine and anesthesia training respectively. She is associate editor, medical humanities, for *BMJ* and poetry editor for *Journal of Medical Humanities*. She co-directs the scholarly concentration in biomedical ethics and medical humanities, teaches creative writing for medical students and strives to create an environment at the medical school to encourage creative exploration, collaboration and scholarly work in medical humanities. She is a founding member of Stanford Pegasus Physician Writers. Her poetry appears in numerous journals and anthologies, and she is the author of *The Mailbox*, a story about post-traumatic stress disorder in Vietnam veterans.

Jasna Krmpotić Schwind, RN, BA, MEd, PhD, is Associate Professor in the Daphne Cockwell School of Nursing at Ryerson University, Toronto, Ontario. Her program of research focuses on reconstruction of experience within professional and therapeutic relationships in education and practice. Using narrative inquiry, she explores the humanness within person-centred care in education and practice and how these impact the quality of a person's illness experience. To this end, she has adapted a form of narrative reflection she terms narrative reflective process (NRP), a creative self-expression strategy that includes storytelling, metaphor, drawing and creative writing. NRP may be used as both a data collection strategy in research, as well as an implementation tool in practice. Dr. Schwind's areas of research and teaching scholarship include human experience of illness and the humanness of care; professional therapeutic relationships in education and practice involving person-centred care; the reconstruction of personal and professional experiences using the narrative reflective process; metaphors as vehicles for personal and professional understanding of self and other; and narrative inquiry as a qualitative research method for health care professionals.

André Smith is Associate Professor of Sociology at the University of Victoria and a Research Affiliate with its Centre on Aging. He has research interests in the areas of aging, ethnicity and mental health. Dr. Smith's research interests reflect a desire to understand health and illness in relation to their social, institutional and policy contexts.

Louise Terry, PhD, PGCHE, LLB (Hons), FIBMS, is a health care professional (biomedical scientist) of more than 30 years' standing with a law degree and a doctorate in medical law and ethics. Her thesis, *Saying No: Withholding and Withdrawing Medical Treatment*, explored how consultant doctors make decisions. She is a member of the Clinical Ethics Committee at St. Christopher's Hospice (founded by Dame Cicely Saunders). She has taught ethics and law to undergraduate and postgraduate health and social care students at London South Bank University since 1998. Louise has received three teaching research fellowships and been twice nominated for national teaching fellowships. In addition to using the arts and humanities in her ethics teaching, Louise was an early pioneer of e-learning, using it to link registered nurses with their counterparts at the University of Washington, Bothell, United States (where she is an international affiliate faculty member) so that students could explore the impact of health care culture on care. In 2010, she edited a book of poems on health and social care values written by London South Bank University students and staff. Her current research includes exploring the development of nursing wisdom as well as researching the continuing professional development of nurses.

Janice Valdez is an interdisciplinary artist, practitioner, facilitator and educational consultant. She has extensive experience in the field of applied creative arts and has facilitated educational drama workshops for youth, adults and their service-providers.

Marlessa Wesolowski is Artist in Residence at St. Paul's Hospital, Saskatoon, Saskatchewan, where she facilitates innovative approaches to working with patients and their families, community youth and health care professionals through the holistic potential of the creative arts. Marlessa's research and educational interests include indigenous cultures, arts in community health and holistic, humanistic-existential philosophies. She is presently completing her BFA at the University of Saskatchewan.

John J. Guiney Yallop is a parent, a partner and a poet. Dr. Guiney Yallop's research includes poetic inquiry, narrative inquiry, autoethnography and performative social science. He uses these methodologies to explore identities, communities and emotional landscapes. His writing has appeared in literary and scholarly journals. He has presented his work at national and international conferences. Dr. Guiney Yallop is Associate Professor in the School of Education at Acadia University. He lives in Wolfville, Nova Scotia, with his partner, Gary, their daughter, Brittany, and their pets.

Louise Younie, MBChC, DRCOH, DCH, MRCGP, MSc, EdD, is a practicing general practitioner and a clinical senior lecturer with current leadership responsibility in GP tutor faculty development as well as for delivering a variety of undergraduate medical-education courses. She has been pioneering and developing the field of arts-based inquiry in undergraduate medical education for the past 10 years, with an MSc and EdD in this field. She embraces the arts within both her clinical and her educational practice, using the arts educationally to stimulate dialogue, reflection and collaborative learning with medical students. She has found the arts to be an excellent vehicle for student-centred transformative learning, practitioner development and engagement with patients' lived experience and student voices.

Also by Cheryl L. McLean

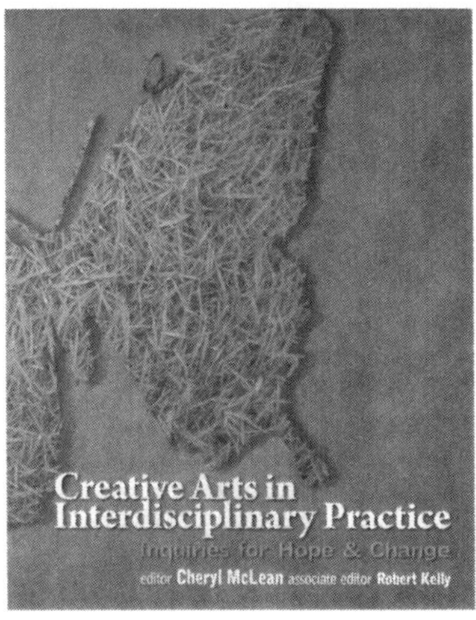

Creative Arts in Interdisciplinary Practice: Inquiries for Hope and Change

Edited by Cheryl L. McLean and Robert Kelly

In this collection of creative research in action, leading academics, health researchers, physicians, educators, environmentalists, and artists share how they're using the creative arts in cutting-edge research and in methodologies for health, hope, and change.

9781550593853
$29.95, softcover

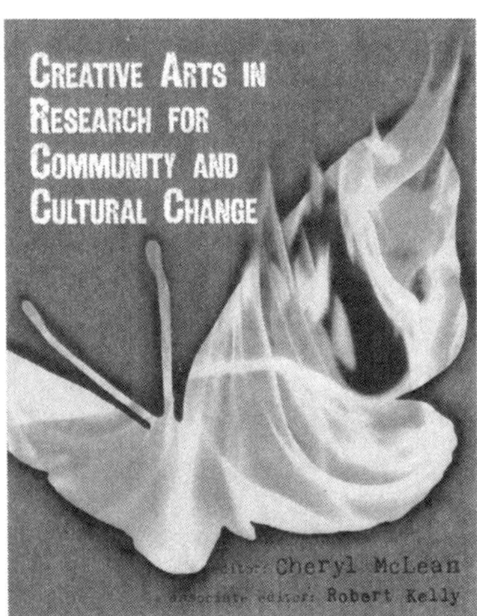

Creative Arts in Research for Community and Cultural Change

Edited by Cheryl L. McLean and Robert Kelly

These articles describe the creative arts in research and practice as a tool for change in communities around the world. They also provide a starting point for creative new approaches in contemporary research leading to social change and democratic justice.

9781550593952
$37.95, softcover